Essential Notes for the FRCS (Urol)

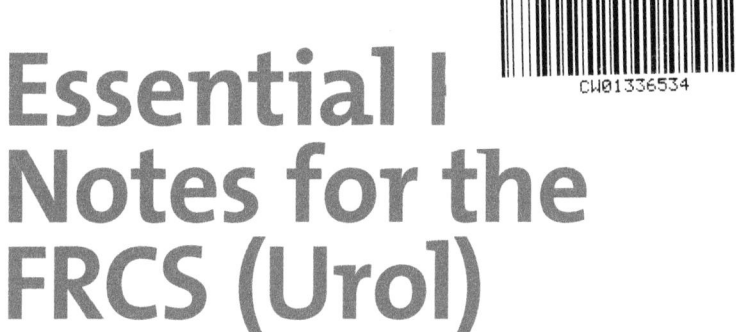

Jack Donati-Bourne

Book 1

Foreword by
Keith Yeates
Gold Medal Winners
Nicholas Rukin
and
Rebecca Tregunna

First published in 2020 by Libri Publishing

Copyright © Jack Donati-Bourne

The right of Jack Donati-Bourne to be identified as the author of this work has been asserted in accordance with the Copyright, Designs and Patents Act, 1988.

ISBN 978-1-911450-70-2

All rights reserved. No part of this publication may be reproduced, stored in any retrieval system or transmitted in any form or by any means, electronic, mechanical, photocopying, recording or otherwise, without the prior written permission of the copyright holder for which application should be addressed in the first instance to the publishers. No liability shall be attached to the author, the copyright holder or the publishers for loss or damage of any nature suffered as a result of reliance on the reproduction of any of the contents of this publication or any errors or omissions in its contents.

A CIP catalogue record for this book is available from The British Library

Cover and Design by Carnegie Publishing

Libri Publishing
Brunel House
Volunteer Way
Faringdon
Oxfordshire
SN7 7YR

Tel: +44 (0)845 873 3837

www.libripublishing.co.uk

CONTENTS

ACKNOWLEDGEMENTS	V
FOREWORD: NICHOLAS J RUKIN	VII
FOREWORD: REBECCA TREGUNNA	IX
INTRODUCTION	XI
GLOSSARY OF ABBREVIATIONS	XIII
STATION 1: UROLOGICAL ONCOLOGY 1	1
STATION 2: UROLOGICAL ONCOLOGY 2	79
STATION 3: PAEDIATRIC UROLOGY	169
STATION 4: EMERGENCY UROLOGY	241
ANSWERS TO MCQS	307
STATION 1: UROLOGICAL ONCOLOGY 1	307
STATION 2: UROLOGICAL ONCOLOGY 2	308
STATION 3: PAEDIATRIC UROLOGY	309
STATION 4: EMERGENCY UROLOGY	310

ACKNOWLEDGEMENTS

Taking on and passing the FRCS (Urol) is a team effort – I would never have managed on my own.

I wish to thank my "triple-A" rated revision group – Anthony (Noah), Adeel (Khan) and Ahmed (Kodera). They taught, supported and accompanied me throughout the long journey to the end, I hope I was able to help you as much as you all helped me – indeed we still have our FRCS (Urol) WhatsApp group to this day.

Many colleagues kindly gifted their precious time to help with exam advice and viva practice, I hope I have included all of them. Thank you to Rupesh Bhatt, Anand Dhanasekaran, Herman Fernando, David Muthuveloe, Praveen Pillai, Philip Polson, Hosam Serag, William Taylor, Rebecca Tregunna and Dan Wood.

Finally, I am very grateful to the authors of "Viva Practice for the FRCS (Urol) and Postgraduate Urology Examinations" (Arya M et al.) – your book was of great assistance and was the only light I had to guide me through the exam darkness. I hope my book will now complement yours and together we can support FRCS (Urol) candidates in the future.

For the production of this book I wish to thank Roger Amos, Celia Cozens and John Sivak from Libri Publishing for having faith in me and my project at the beginning and providing fantastic support throughout the publication process.

For support during particularly difficult exam times I am indebted to Harry, Darryl, Suleiman, Jessica, Juan and Aunty Shanaz.

I dedicate this book to my dad – I hope he would have been proud of me if he could read it, to my mum – to whom I owe simply everything, and to Shamah – thank you for teaching me about what really matters in life, I love you.

FOREWORD

Postgraduate examinations can be a tough time for trainees and their loved ones. When to start revising, what to start revising first and where to find the relevant information are common barriers to revision. Many textbooks are available which contain the in-depth knowledge about specifics, but the majority of these cannot be learnt from cover to cover for fellowship exams. This book enables the reader to start the preparation for the FRCS (Urol) in a structured and logical manner. Although written specifically for the inter-collegiate fellowship of the Royal Colleges of Surgeons FRCS (Urol) examination, this text will be of use to all trainees undertaking fellowship examinations.

Hopefully, the FRCS (Urol) exam will be your last major hurdle before completing your training and moving on to the next step of your career as a consultant urological surgeon. People approach the exam in many different ways, each specific to their individual learning style, and by this stage of your career you know what works best for you. I would advise you to stick with what has worked previously, as it has worked well for you to get to this stage in your professional life.

I have always advocated that your entire specialist training is your consultant job interview. You have been assessed on a daily basis until this point, from ward rounds to the operating theatre and including non-technical skills. The FRCS (Urol) is the next step in this continued assessment. The same key factors are being examined, this time by examiners rather than your trainer. This is your time to shine, show your knowledge and prove to the examiners that you are a safe, knowledgeable and independent year one consultant urological surgeon. Treat the exam as your chance to demonstrate to your peers all you have learned over the years. Some things are straight forward facts, ciprofloxacin is a fluoroquinolone which works by inhibiting DNA gyrase, others are more considered and a balanced answer stating your personal opinion having weighed up the literature is the correct approach (e.g. screening for prostate cancer).

I would advise you to look at the exam positively, it is your only opportunity to fully understand and learn the basic science, physiology, pathophysiology, pharmacology, anatomy and evidence basis for the things you do in your daily practice. For example, we all would aim to give mitomycin-C post initial TURBT, but do you really know why? To say it reduces recurrence is true, but to deliver the Sylvester meta-analysis quoting a relative risk reduction of 39%, absolute risk reduction of 12% and NNT of 7 for non-muscle invasive disease should be the aim. Incorporating this into your daily ward round and post-op information to the patient will reinforce the evidence, but more importantly it enables the patient to make an informed choice. Learning is lifelong and you will find many things you learn for the fellowship exam will become vital in independent practice.

The two parts of the exam require different learning and exam practice. MCQs need to be practiced, and there are multiple learning resources available online or in-print. Practice technique, practice interpretation and practice quick facts. Don't neglect common things such as TNM staging in favour of the minutiae of Retzius sparing robotic prostatectomy. Part two focuses on the delivery of knowledge. Practising oral exams with colleagues, fellow trainees and trainers is vital in preparing delivery of facts. Get used to speaking loudly and confidently. Look at the examiner, engage them like you would on a post-take ward round or in clinic. Show knowledge, insight and appreciate both patient and pathological factors. The key is to demonstrate safe independent urological practice and not to recite a textbook. Patients can be complex, with multiple confounding factors that do not fit a 'gold standard' answer but more a discussion of several suitable treatment options.

My research professor commonly quoted Erwin Rommel, a German field marshal: "time spent in reconnaissance is seldom wasted". This quote is equally applicable to fellowship examinations, the more time spent on revision and background work will only amplify your knowledge and enhance your exam performance.

Good luck, work hard, prepare around the syllabus and make sure you give your best performance on the exam day. Nerves get us all, and if you feel stressed on the day just remember to be safe and sensible with your answers. Show maturity in your thinking, rationale and delivery. You will become a better, all-rounded urological surgeon from this exam and you will one day look back on the experience as a positive one. I promise you that!

Nicholas J Rukin
MBChB MD FRCSEd (Urol) FRACS (Urol)

Consultant Urological Surgeon
Metro North Hospital and Health Service, Brisbane, Australia

FOREWORD

Following at least seven years of postgraduate training and achieving an Outcome 1 at your ST5 Annual Review of Competence Progression you will embark on the final hurdle, and hopefully your final ever examination: the FRCS (Urol). You will dig out the notes made on scraps of paper and pharmaceutical company notepads from the years of deanery teaching sessions you have attended only to realise the lecture that the ST3 gave on benign prostatic hypertrophy was written in haste the night before and barely covers the basics. You will then decide that you must know everything about urology and try to read the most comprehensive of texts: Campbell-Walsh-Wein from cover to cover, only to panic when you realise it has taken a week to read the first four chapters and there are at least a hundred and fifty to go. This is when the real panic sets in.

There is no doubt that the FRCS (Urol) examination is a daunting task. Urology is a rapidly evolving field and the archive of revision notes and multiple choice question banks that are shared amongst trainees, although helpful, are out of date and do not cover entire swathes of the curriculum. Section 1 of the examination comprises two papers of single best answer and extended matching questions undertaken in your local Pearson Vue Centre alongside people taking their driving theory test, which can be both distracting as well as embarrassing as you try to shield the seventeen-year-old provisional drivers (who enter and leave every twenty minutes) from the pictures of Peyronie's disease flashing up on your screen. Section 2 is potentially no less embarrassing as it consists of eight separate 20-minute viva stations and for most doctors this will be the first time they have ever had to undertake this sort of cross-examination: a truly harrowing prospect.

There are plenty of excellent revision and mock viva practice courses aimed at section 2; my advice is to attend all of them if you can. Start saving as they can be expensive, but taking the exam twice is even more costly and the chances are that your family will not thank you for having to take even more time off to revise. One thing that candidates who have completed the examination will say is that although the viva is intimidating, it is fair. Examiners are looking for a safe, day one consultant who they would be happy to employ and leave in charge of their patients over the weekend. References to data from trials and other journal articles are certainly not necessary, (there are a few exceptions; the BAUS revision course will cover the important papers you should know) but if you are pushing for the Keith Yeates Gold Medal they can help to justify why you would offer a patient a certain treatment. The most important aspect of this section is your interaction with examiners. Practice viva stations regularly with your colleagues and try not to come across as an under-confident registrar. Your examiners are soon to be your colleagues so have a professional discussion with them, (try to) relax, ensure you have a logical thought process and speak slowly and clearly.

Section 1 in my opinion is actually more difficult. It is far more arbitrary than section 2 and there is a real time pressure during the test. I suggest that you start to make notes six months before the examination and really knuckle down when you have three months to go. Practising multiple-choice questions is useful but to get a real foundation of knowledge Jack Donati-Bourne has done a lot of the hard work for you by writing this comprehensive book of revision notes. This publication covers the entire spectrum of the intercollegiate speciality examination curriculum in a succinct, logical way, ensuring that information pertinent to *both* sections of the examination is presented. This means no more panic about which texts to use now that this pre-eminent resource is readily available.

Revision can be hard, laborious and lonely. Try not to be overwhelmed, work hard but take plenty of rest breaks (I completed several seasons of RuPaul's Drag Race), have a close circle of friends with whom you can both laugh and vociferate, and take time for yourself and your family. I would also actively encourage you to take a couple of weeks of leave before each section to seriously revise with minimal distraction (delete Facebook, TikTok and Instagram from your phone now).

Remember at the end of this period you will be more knowledgeable than you ever have been, and it really is a good feeling when you can present to a patient or colleague the objective evidence behind a treatment option.

To quote William Shakespeare: *"Ignorance is the curse of God; knowledge the wing wherewith we fly to heaven"* and to urologically paraphrase RuPaul Charles: *"Good Luck, and don't balls it up"*!

Rebecca Tregunna
MBBS BSc (Hons) FRCS (Urol)

Pelvic Oncology Senior Robotic Fellow
Eastbourne District General Hospital, East Sussex, UK

INTRODUCTION

Thank you for choosing my book!

I do sincerely hope you will find it useful and that above all it helps you pass the FRCS (Urol) exam, which is an important milestone in your career as a urologist and, for many, the last exam in a long series of assessments dating back from medical school.

When preparing for the FRCS (Urol) I often felt that I did not have a clear compass for my revision. Resources for the exam were very scarce, and I was never entirely sure that I was focusing my time and efforts in the right direction. The FRCS (Urol) is stressful enough as it is, and I wanted to take that stress of the "unknown" away for you – and that was the impetus to write this book. I believe that if you read this book in full and use it alongside your other resources, it will serve as a really helpful guide for your revision.

I thought I would briefly share a few of my own reflections with you, mainly to provide encouragement and reassurance that you are not alone if you are feeling stressed, tired and nervous about this exam.

The FRCS (Urol) exam is a tough challenge – it is a taxing exam in itself, but also the time when most take it naturally tends to coincide with a phase in life which for many of us is very busy. Many of you may be newly married or moving in with your partners, expecting or looking after young children, buying a new home… not to mention working a busy hospital job, learning how to operate on patients and who knows maybe even trying to maintain a semblance of a social life!

Furthermore like any skill in life, taking exams is easier with practice and now that you have decided to sit the FRCS (Urol) you may find it has been many years since you last sat down and took time out of your life to prepare for an exam.

Personally I found this to be the biggest challenge of the FRCS (Urol), and whilst there are many things in life we cannot change or control, there are some pieces of advice which I believe are helpful.

Firstly, plan ahead and choose the right moment to take the FRCS (Urol). I strongly recommend you fully focus on the aim to pass both parts first time, but in so doing you have to accept that 6 to 7 months of your life have to be set aside to take the exam and are effectively a write-off. Time the exam such that if possible, you avoid juggling other important commitments such as moving house, having babies or planning weddings. You are much better off nailing the exam first time rather than giving it less than 100% effort and finding yourself having to repeat a section, with all the added stress this entails and the prolonged time with the FRCS (Urol) hanging over your (and your family's) head.

Secondly, do not try to tackle this exam on your own. Speak to senior colleagues who have recently taken the exam (you will find there is always a folder full of exam material saved on somebody's hard drive going round). Form positive connections and revision groups with peers taking the exam with you – group revision is absolutely essential, particularly for the viva. You will not succeed in the viva if you do not practise regularly in your group.

Ensure your family is well aware of the upcoming challenge and that you need their support during this stressful time. Remember we are stronger together.

Lastly, do not worry. The exam is not easy, but it is fair! If you set aside plenty of time, put the right amount of effort and use the correct resources, you will pass. And even if you don't – well, there are many consultants who had to retake it and they are just fine and very successful now!

There are positives – although I had many late nights, tired mornings and missed social events, what I can say is that for probably the first time in my life I found the revision enjoyable. I realised that all the knowledge was directly relevant to my future practice as a urologist. I was finally understanding the rationale and evidence behind my daily clinical practice rather than relying on transcended knowledge from a more senior colleague telling me "this is how it should be done". Finally, when I came out the other end of the FRCS (Urol), I felt so much more confident in hospital and in looking after my patients, which is a priceless and enduring satisfaction to have.

I do wish you all the best with the FRCS (Urol). Good luck!

Jack Donati-Bourne (2020)

GLOSSARY OF ABBREVIATIONS

AAST – American Association for the Surgery of Trauma
AC – assisted conception
ACT – α1 anti-chymotrypsin
ACTH – adreno-corticotropic hormone
AD – autonomic dysreflexia
ADH – anti-diuretic hormone
ADT – androgen deprivation therapy
AFP – alpha feto-protein
AKI – acute kidney injury
ADPKD – autosomal dominant polycystic kidney disease
ALP – alkaline phosphatase
ALPP – abdominal leak point pressure
AMG – α2 macro globulin
AML – angiomyolipoma
ANP – atrial natriuretic peptide
AP – antero-posterior
APD – antero-posterior diameter
APC – adenomatous polyposis coli
ARCD – acquired renal cystic disease
ARR – absolute risk reduction
ASAP – atypical small acinar proliferation
AS – active surveillance
AUA – American Urology Association
AUR – acute urinary retention
AUS – artificial urinary sphincter
BAPU – British Association of Paediatric Urologists
BCI – bladder contractility index
BMD – bone mineral density
BOO – bladder outlet obstruction
BOOI – bladder outlet obstruction index
BPH – benign prostatic hyperplasia
BPS – bladder pain syndrome
BTB – blood-testis barrier
BTx – brachytherapy
BXO – balanitis xerotica obliterans
CAH – congenital adrenal hyperplasia
CAIS – Complete Androgen Insensitivity Syndrome
CAP – continuous antibiotic prophylaxis

CBAVD – congenital bilateral absence of vas deferens
CCG – clinical commissioning group
CCI – Charlson comorbidity index
cCMP – cyclic guanosine monophosphate
CF – cystic fibrosis
CFU – colony forming units
CI – confidence interval
CIS – carcinoma in-situ
CKD – chronic kidney disease
CMV – cytomegalovirus
CN – cytoreductive nephrectomy
CNS – central nervous system
COPD – chronic obstructive pulmonary disease
CPPS – chronic pelvic pain syndrome
CRP – C-reactive protein
CRPC – castrate resistant prostate cancer
CSS – cancer specific survival
CT – computed tomography
CT TAP – computed tomography of thorax abdomen and pelvis
CTU – computed tomography urogram
CVA – cerebrovascular accident
CXR – chest x-ray
DCE – dynamic contrast enhanced
DetSD – detrusor sphincter dyssynergia
DEXA – dual energy absorptiometry scan
DHT – dihydrotestosterone
DLPP – detrusor leak point pressure
DMSA – dimercaptosuccinic acid
DNA – deoxyribonucleic acid
DO – detrusor overactivity
DRE – digital rectal examination
DSD – disorder of sexual differentiation
DSNB – dynamic sentinel node biopsy
DW-MRI – diffusion-weighted magnetic resonance imaging
EAU – European Association of Urology
EBRT – external beam radiotherapy
ECG – electro-cardiogram
ECOG – Eastern Cooperative Oncology Group
ED – erectile dysfunction
EDTA – ethylene diamine tetra acetic acid
EMA – European Medicines Agency

EMRT – emergency medical response team
EORTC – European Organisation for Research and Treatment of Cancer
EPLND – extended pelvic lymph node dissection
EPN – emphysematous pyelonephritis
EPO – erythropoietin
EPR – extra-peritoneal rupture
ERSPC – European Randomised Study of Screening for Prostate Cancer
ESRF – end-stage renal failure
ESWL – extra-corporeal shockwave lithotripsy
ETS – E26 Transformation Specific
FBC – full blood count
FDG – fluorodeoxyglucose
FNA – fine-needle aspiration
FSH – follicle stimulating hormone
FUD – female urethral diverticulum
FVC – frequency volume chart
f/T PSA – free to total prostate specific antigen
GA – general anaesthesia
GAG – glycosaminoglycans
GCNIS – germ cell neoplasia in situ
GCS – Glasgow coma scale
GCT – germ cell tumour
GFR – glomerular filtration rate
GnRH – gonadotropin-releasing hormone
GS – Gram stain
GUCG – Genito-Urinary Cancer Group
HDL – high-density lipoprotein
HEPA – high efficiency particulate air
HGPIN – high grade prostatic intra-epithelial neoplasia
HIFU – high-intensity focused ultrasound
HIV – human immunodeficiency virus
HK – human kallikrein
HLRCC – hereditary leiomyomatosis and renal cell carcinoma
HPCRU – high pressure chronic retention of urine
HPF – high-powered field
HPG – hypothalamo-pituitary-gonadal
HPRC – hereditary papillary renal cell carcinoma
HPV – human papilloma virus
HU – Hounsfield unit
ICCS – International Children's Continence Society
ICD – implantable cardioverter defibrillator

ICIQ-UI – International Consultation on Incontinence Questionnaire
ICS – International Continence Society
ICSI – intra-cytoplasmic sperm injection
IDO – idiopathic detrusor overactivity
IGF – insulin growth factor
IHD – ischaemic heart disease
IHT – intermittent hormone therapy
IM – intra-muscular
INR – international normalised ratio
IPR – intra-peritoneal rupture
IPSS – International Prostate Symptom Score
ISC – intermittent self catheterisation
ISD – intermittent self dilatation
ISUP – International Society of Urological Pathology
ITGCN – intra-tubular germ cell neoplasia
ITU – intensive therapy unit
IUI – intra-uterine insemination
IV – intra-venous
IVF – in-vitro fertilisation
KSS – kidney sparing surgery
kD – kilo Dalton
LASER – Light Amplification by Stimulated Emission of Radiation
LDL – low-density lipoprotein
LFT – liver function tests
LH – luteinising hormone
LHRH – luteinising hormone releasing hormone
LLN – lower limit of normal
LN – lymph node
LND – lymph node dissection
LPS – lower pole stone
LTC – long term catheter
LUT – lower urinary tract
LUTD – lower urinary tract dysfunction
LUTS – lower urinary tract symptoms
LVI – lymphovascular invasion
MAB – maximum androgen blockade
MAG3 – mercapto acetyltriglycine
MAP – mean arterial pressure
MCDK – multi-cystic dysplastic kidney
mCRPC – metastatic castrate resistant prostate cancer
MCUG – micturating cysto-urethrogram

MDP – methylene diphosphonate
MDRD – Modification of Diet in Renal Disease study
MDT – multi-disciplinary team
MET – medical expulsive therapy
MHRA – Medicines and Healthcare products Regulatory Agency
MHz – mega Hertz
MIBG – metaiodobenzylguanidine
MIS – Mullerian inhibiting substance
mPCa – metastatic prostate cancer
MRU – magnetic resonance (MR) urogram
MV – mega voltage
mL – millilitre
MNE – monosymptomatic nocturnal enuresis
mpMRI – multi-parametric magnetic resonance imaging
mRCC – metastatic renal cell carcinoma
MRI – magnetic resonance imaging
MS – multiple sclerosis
MSU – mid-stream urine (culture)
MUI – mixed urinary incontinence
NA – noradrenaline
NAAT – nucleic acid amplification test
NC – neoadjuvant chemotherapy
NCCT – non-contrast computed tomography
Nd – neodymium
NDO – neurogenic detrusor overactivity
ng – nanogram
NHS – National Health Service
NICE – National Institute of Clinical Excellence
NIDDK – National Institute of Diabetes, Digestive and Kidney Diseases
NNT – number needed to treat
NO – nitric oxide
NPV – negative predictive value
NS – nerve sparing
NSAID – non-steroidal anti-inflammatory drug
NSGCT – non-seminomatous germ cell tumour
NVH – non-visible haematuria
OAB – overactive bladder
OD – once daily
OS – overall survival
PAE – prostate artery embolization
PCa – prostate cancer

PCNL – percutaneous nephrolithotomy
PDD – photo dynamic diagnosis
PDE5i – phosphodiesterase-5 inhibitor
PDGF – platelet-derived growth factor
PET – positron emission tomography
PID – pelvic inflammatory disease
PIRADS – Prostate Imaging Reporting and Data System
PFE – pelvic floor exercises
PFMT – pelvic floor muscle training
PFS – progression free survival
PFUDD – pelvic fracture posterior urethral distraction defect
PN – partial nephrectomy
PO – per oral
POP – pelvic organ prolapse
PPS – prostate pain syndrome
PPV – patent processus vaginalis
PR – per rectum
PSA – prostate specific antigen
PSAD – prostate specific antigen density
PSADT – prostate specific antigen doubling time
PSATZD – prostate specific antigen transitional zone density
PSAV – prostate specific antigen velocity
PSMA – prostate specific membrane antigen
PTFE – polytetrafluoroethane
PTH – parathyroid hormone
PTNS – posterior tibial nerve stimulation
PUJ – pelviureteric junction
PUJO – pelviureteric junction obstruction
PUNLMP – papillary urothelial neoplasm of low malignant potential
PUV – posterior urethral valves
PVD – peripheral vascular disease
PVR – post-void residual
QDS – quarter die sumendum (four times daily)
QOL – quality of life
qSOFA – quick sepsis-related organ failure assessment
RCC – renal cell carcinoma
RCT – randomised controlled trial
RFA – radiofrequency ablation
RN – radical nephrectomy
RNA – ribonucleic acid
RNU – radical nephroureterectomy

RP – radical prostatectomy
RR – relative risk
RTA – renal tubular acidosis
RTB – renal tumour biopsy
RTC – road traffic collision
RTx – radiotherapy
RU – retrograde urethrogram
rUTI – recurrent urinary tract infection
SCC – spinal cord compression
SCCa – squamous cell carcinoma
SCI – spinal cord injury
SFR – stone-free rate
SNM – sacral neuromodulation
SOFA – sequential organ failure assessment
SPC – suprapubic catheter
SPECT – single-photon emission computed tomography
sPSA – super-sensitive prostate specific antigen
SSRI – selective serotonin reuptake inhibitor
STI – sexually transmitted infection
SUI – stress urinary incontinence
TB – tuberculosis
TC – testicular cancer
Tc – technetium
TCC – transitional cell carcinoma
TDS – ter die sumendum (three times daily)
TENS – trans-cutaneous electrical nerve stimulation
TESE – testicular sperm extraction
TIN – testicular intra-epithelial neoplasia
TMPRSS2 – trans-membrane protease serine 2
TOT – trans-obturator tape
TPN – total parenteral nutrition
TRUS – trans-rectal ultrasound
TSG – tumour suppressor gene
TUIP – trans-urethral incision of prostate
TURBT – trans-urethral resection of bladder tumour
TURED – trans-urethral resection of ejaculatory ducts
TURP – trans-urethral resection of prostate
TVT – trans-vaginal tape
UDS – urodynamics
UDT – undescended testis
UE – urea and electrolytes

ULN – upper limit of normal
URS – ureteroscopy
US – ultrasound
USA – United States of America
UTUC – upper tract urothelial cancer
UUI – urge urinary incontinence
VEGF – vascular endothelial growth factor
VH – visible haematuria
VHL – Von-Hippel Lindau syndrome
VIP – vaso-active intestinal peptide
VLPP – Valsalva leak point pressure
VTE – venous thrombo-embolism
VUDS – video urodynamics
VUR – vesico-ureteric reflux
VVF – vesicovaginal fistula
WHO – World Health Organisation
WLE – wide local excision
WW – watchful waiting
XGP – xanthogranulomatous pyelonephritis
YAG – yttrium aluminium garnet
ZA – zoledronic acid
5AR – 5-alpha reductase
5ARIs – 5-alpha reductase inhibitors
5-FU – 5-fluorouracil

STATION 1
UROLOGICAL ONCOLOGY 1

HAEMATURIA

NON-MUSCLE INVASIVE BLADDER CANCER

MUSCLE-INVASIVE BLADDER CANCER

RENAL CANCER

UPPER TRACT UROTHELIAL CANCER

CONTENTS

HAEMATURIA 7
  DEFINITIONS 7
    NON-VISIBLE HAEMATURIA 7
  CAUSES 8
  NICE GUIDANCE (2015) 9
  INVESTIGATIONS 9
    URINE CYTOLOGY 10
    PHOTODYNAMIC DIAGNOSTIC (PDD) CYSTOSCOPY 11
  NEPHROLOGY REFERRAL 12
    NEPHROLOGICAL CAUSES OF HAEMATURIA 12

NON-MUSCLE INVASIVE BLADDER CANCER 14
  EPIDEMIOLOGY 14
  RISK FACTORS 14
  PATHOLOGY 14
    CARCINOMA-IN-SITU (CIS) 15
    SQUAMOUS CELL CARCINOMA 15
    ADENOCARCINOMA 16
    PRE-MALIGNANT LESIONS 16
    INVESTIGATIONS 16
    TRANS-URETHRAL RESECTION OF BLADDER TUMOUR 16
    SECOND RESECTION 17
  GRADING 18
  STAGING 19
  RISK STRATIFICATION 20
  MANAGEMENT 22
    MITOMYCIN-C 22
    BCG THERAPY 23
    RE-RESECTION 25
    RADICAL CYSTECTOMY 26
    G3PT1 DISEASE MANAGEMENT 26
    CIS MANAGEMENT 26
    RECURRENT NMIBC (LOW RISK) 26

STATION 1: UROLOGICAL ONCOLOGY 1

NICE (2020) MANAGEMENT SUMMARY	27
MUSCLE-INVASIVE BLADDER CANCER	**28**
OVERVIEW	28
ASSESSMENT	28
IMAGING	29
CT SCAN	29
MRI SCAN	29
PROGNOSTIC EVALUATION	30
TREATMENT	32
TREATMENT FAILURE OF NMIBC	32
NEO-ADJUVANT CHEMOTHERAPY	32
ADJUVANT CHEMOTHERAPY	33
RADICAL EXTERNAL BEAM RADIOTHERAPY (EBRT)	33
RADICAL CYSTECTOMY (RC)	34
COMPLICATIONS AFTER RC	36
URINARY DIVERSION	38
EBRT VS. RC	40
PARTIAL CYSTECTOMY (PC)	40
METASTATIC DISEASE	40
MANAGEMENT	41
CHEMOTHERAPY	41
URACHAL TUMOUR	41
RENAL CANCER	**42**
EPIDEMIOLOGY	42
RISK FACTORS	42
HEREDITARY CONDITIONS	42
ANGIOMYOLIPOMA	44
DIAGNOSIS	46
PRESENTATION	46
IMAGING	46
CT UROGRAM	46
MR-UROGRAM	47
BOSNIAK CLASSIFICATION OF RENAL CYSTS	47
RENAL TUMOUR BIOPSY	48

STAGING	49
PROGNOSTIC FACTORS	51
TREATMENT	53
NEPHRON-SPARING SURGERY	53
RADICAL NEPHRECTOMY	57
ACTIVE SURVEILLANCE	58
CRYOSURGERY (CS)	58
RADIO-FREQUENCY ABLATION	59
FOLLOW-UP	59
METASTATIC RCC	60
BENIGN RENAL MASSES	62
POLYCYSTIC KIDNEY DISEASE	62
ACQUIRED RENAL CYSTIC DISEASE	62
MULTI-CYSTIC DYSPLASTIC KIDNEY	62
MULTI-LOCULAR CYST (CYSTIC NEPHROMA)	63
ONCOCYTOMA	63
UPPER TRACT UROTHELIAL CANCER	**64**
EPIDEMIOLOGY	64
RISK FACTORS	64
DIAGNOSIS	64
SYMPTOMS	64
IMAGING	65
CYTOLOGY	65
DIAGNOSTIC URETEROSCOPY	65
STAGING	65
TREATMENT	66
KIDNEY SPARING SURGERY	66
RADICAL NEPHROURETERECTOMY	67
CHEMO-RADIO THERAPY	68
FOLLOW-UP	68
METASTATIC DISEASE	68
REFERENCES	**69**
UROLOGICAL ONCOLOGY 1 MCQS	**73**

HAEMATURIA

DEFINITIONS

Visible haematuria (VH) (formerly known as "gross" or "macroscopic")
- it is the most common presenting symptom of bladder cancer
- along with storage urinary symptoms occurs in 20% patients with CIS or bladder cancer

Non-visible haematuria (NVH):
- symptomatic NVH (s-NVH) i.e. in the presence of lower urinary tract symptoms
- asymptomatic NVH (a-NVH)

Table 1 – Definition of NVH according to differing guidelines: [1]

AUA + Campbell's	3+ RBCs per high-powered field
Nephrology	>5 RBCs per micro litre

NON-VISIBLE HAEMATURIA

Trace haematuria is considered negative.

No distinction is made between haemolysed and non-haemolysed dipstick-positive urine.

Prevalence in 2.5% of men and 10% of women

Transient contamination from vigorous exercise, sexual intercourse or menstruation

Overall 10% of patients with NVH will have urological malignancy.

Table 2 – the NVH on urine dipstick in relation to number of RBCs per high-powered field [1]

Dipstick Result	RBCs per high-powered Field
+	1–10
++	10–40
+++	40–100

Mechanism of Action

Urine dipstick for NVH relies on oxidation of a chromogen by the peroxidase activity of haemoglobin, resulting in colour change on strip which is compared to known standards.

False negative – samples sent from community or GP have a high false-negative rate due to red-cell lysis in transit.

False positive – occurs in presence of myoglobinuria, bacterial peroxides, povidone, menstruation.

CAUSES

Table 3 – summary of causes of VH

Stones	Kidney, ureter, bladder
Infection	Bacterial, mycobacterial (TB), parasitic (schistosomiasis)
Oncological	Renal, ureteric, bladder, prostate, urethral
Benign	BPH
(Nephrological)	(further listed below)

Haematuria in BPH

Aetiological causes include:
- Increased prostatic vascularity due to higher micro vessel density in hyperplastic prostatic tissue
- Elevated expression of VEGF

BPH-related haematuria can be treated with 5-alpha reductase inhibitors as first-line (emergency TURP or prostatic artery embolization are subsequent options)
- Success rate of 90%

Finasteride will decrease VEGF expression, micro vessel density and prostatic blood flow. [2]

Screening for Bladder Cancer

Studies by Britton et al. (1992) [3] and Messing et al. (2006) [4] screened thousands of patients via dipstick test, finding 15–20% had NVH.

However the false-positive rate was 90% which would therefore yield a prohibitively high number of patients for investigation.

Khadra et al. (2000) reviewed almost 2000 haematuria clinic patients, finding urinary tract malignancy in 13% (9.4% of NVH referrals and 24.2% in VH referrals). [5]

NICE GUIDANCE (2015)

NICE (2015) released guidance for "Suspected cancer: recognition and referral" [7] for haematuria under bladder cancer category – it is essential to memorise this for the exam.

Table 4 – NICE (2015) Guidelines for referral of haematuria

Aged > 45 years	• unexplained VH without UTI • VH that persists or recurs after UTI treatment
Aged > 60 years	• unexplained NVH + (raised WCC or dysuria)
Non-urgent bladder cancer referral	Aged > 60 years with new unexplained recurrent UTIs

Criteria used to devise the NICE guideline for NVH was drawn from a study by Price et al. (2014) undertaken in General Practice.

Almost 5000 patients with known bladder cancer were compared with > 20,000 matched controls, to estimate the PPV for bladder cancer of various factors.

PPV was highest for raised WCC (PPV = 3.9) and dysuria (4.5).

INVESTIGATIONS

Ideally eligible patients should be referred to a one-stop haematuria clinic.

History:
- onset, duration, associated symptoms
- past medical history, drug history
- smoking status and occupational exposure to carcinogens

Examination:
- abdominal examination, external genitalia, pelvic examination in women

MSU and Urine Cytology

Blood tests:
- FBC / UE / clotting screen
- PSA to be considered if VH, LUTS or ED (NICE Guidance 2015)

Flexible cystoscopy

Imaging:
- USS and / or CT-urogram

URINE CYTOLOGY

Best sample is mid-morning (not early morning as these samples provide degenerate specimens).

Whole stream analysis is preferable, as mid-stream is the most acellular fraction.

Catheter specimens can be analysed but may have undergone changes, saline washouts will need to be centrifuged and fixed in formalin.

Analysis must be fast, if prolonged delay expected refrigerate the sample or fix with 50% alcohol.

High specificity of cytology is 95%.

For high-grade tumours the sensitivity is 90% and therefore is most useful in this context, however it is only 10% for low-grade tumours.

Positive predictive value (PPV) for cytology is highest due to low number of false positives.

Alternative Urinary Markers for Urothelial Carcinoma

Urine cytology has a weak sensitivity for detecting low-grade urothelial carcinomas and therefore novel markers have been developed, although these are not yet accepted in clinical diagnosis or follow-up in current guidelines.

Nuclear-matrix protein 22 (NMP 22)

Bladder tumour associated antigen (BTA stat)

- identifies the over-production of the complement protective peptide complement factor H related protein in the urine

Telomerase
- over expressed in many cancers and can be detected in the urine with Telomerase Repeat Amplification (TRAP)

Urovysion test
- utilises fluorescent in-situ hybridisation (FISH) to test for aneuploidy of chromosomes 3, 7, 17 and loss of 9p21

Positive Cytology, Normal Other Haematuria Investigations

Undertake CT-urogram if not already done.

Consent the patient for:
- rigid cystoscopy and bladder biopsies of trigone, right and left lateral walls, posterior wall and dome, looking for carcinoma-in-situ (CIS)
- consider bilateral retrograde studies and ureteroscopy

In men consider prostatic urethra biopsies when no tumour seen in the bladder.

PHOTODYNAMIC DIAGNOSTIC (PDD) CYSTOSCOPY

Relies on the molecular handling of 5-aminolevulinic acid (5-ALA) by tumour cells

Procedure:
- instil 5-ALA into bladder > 1 hour prior to cystoscopy (taken up by urothelium)
- 5-ALA is converted to protoporphyrin which is preferentially taken up by malignant cells
- when blue light (375–440 nm wavelength) illuminates bladder, areas of red fluorescence from abnormal mucosa will light up surrounding normal bladder mucosa
- any resection of abnormal blue light area should be undertaken with white light, then at final check under blue light the affected area should no long be visible

No benefit on disease-specific survival rates has been demonstrated to date.

PHOTO Trial:

- underway as a multi-centre randomised trial comparing PDD guided bladder tumour resection with standard white-light in patient newly diagnosed NMIBC
- analysing cost effectiveness and time to recurrence

NEPHROLOGY REFERRAL

Joint Consensus Statement on the Initial Assessment of Haematuria prepared on behalf of the Renal Association and British Association of Urological Surgeons (2008) outlined guidelines for referral to nephrology. [8]

Patients with negative urological investigations need nephrology referral if other factors present:

- declining eGFR by > 10mL / min within last 5 years or > 5 mL / min within last 1 year
- stage 4 or 5 CKD
- significant proteinuria (albumin to creatinine ratio [ACR] > 30mg / mmol)

Consider primary nephrology referral in patients under 40 years of age with NVH considering the risk factors for glomerulonephritis:

- significant proteinuria (albumin to creatinine ratio [ACR] > 30mg / mmol)
- hypertension (BP > 140 / 90)
- eGFR < 60 mL / min

NEPHROLOGICAL CAUSES OF HAEMATURIA

Glomerular Causes:

- *IgA nephropathy* (Berger's disease) involves deposition of IgA after an upper respiratory tract infection, worse if concomitant VH / NVH
- *Alport's syndrome* involves X-linked collagen mutation resulting in nephritis
- *Goodpasture's syndrome* is auto-immune disease where antibodies attack the basement membrane of kidneys resulting in NVH

- *Nephrotic syndrome* results from non-inflammatory injury to the glomerulus, associated with proteinuria, hypoalbuminaemia, hypercholesterolaemia and hyperlipidaemia
- *Henoch-Schonlein purpura* is a systemic vasculitis characterised by deposition of immune complexes containing IgA

Non-glomerular Causes:

- *renal artery stenosis* (when stenosis > 70%)
- *papillary necrosis* is coagulative necrosis of renal papillae due to pyelonephritis, obstructive uropathy, sickle cell, TB, trauma, cirrhosis, analgesic nephropathy, renal vein thrombosis, diabetes (POSTCARD acronym)
- *interstitial nephritis* involves inflammatory infiltrate affecting nephron function

NON-MUSCLE INVASIVE BLADDER CANCER

EPIDEMIOLOGY

7th most common cancer in men, 11th most common in women.

The majority (80%) of patients present with non-muscle invasive disease (Ta, CIS, sub-mucosa T1).

The most common presenting symptom is painless visible haematuria, and the concomitance of irritative lower urinary tract symptoms can suggest presence of CIS.

5% of patients will have metachronous upper-tract TCC.

RISK FACTORS

Smoking — most important risk factor accounting for 50% of cases (increased aromatic amine excretion in urine) with 2–5x increased risk

Age — most commonly diagnosed > 80 years

Occupational — 10% of all cases, from exposure to aromatic amines (paint, dye, petroleum, rubber) and chlorination of drinking water

Inflammation — chronic inflammatory conditions such as schistosomiasis

Drugs — cyclophosphamide (chemotherapy agent to treat haematological cancers)

Radiotherapy — pelvic irradiation to treat cancer can increase risk 2–4x

Genetic — family history not known influence, no clear genetic causes found, although karyotypic changes of chromosomes 9, 17 (p53) & 13 (retinoblastoma loci)

PATHOLOGY

95% of patients with bladder cancer have transitional cell carcinoma (TCC), the remaining have squamous cell carcinoma (SCC) (4%) and adenocarcinoma.

In areas where schistosomiasis is endemic, 75% of bladder cancers are SCC in origin.

Rare bladder cancers include small cell (identical to pulmonary and usually neuroendocrine), sarcomatoid and nested variants.

The most common sarcoma involving the bladder is leiomyosarcoma, which is not associated with smoking history.

pTa low-grade is the most common NMIBC found in approximately 50–70% of such patients, CIS is in 10% of NMIBC and pTa high-grade is rare and likely misclassification.

Tumour spread:
- *haematogenous*, to liver, lung, adrenal gland and bone
- *lymphatic*, iliac and para-aortic lymph nodes
- *implantation*, via direct seeding (e.g. supra-pubic catheterisation)
- *direct invasion*, to prostate, adnexal organs, bowel

CARCINOMA-IN-SITU (CIS)

CIS is a flat, high-grade, non-invasive urothelial carcinoma, easily mistaken for inflammatory lesion if not biopsied (can also occur in upper tract) and is often multi-focal.

CIS cells show a high percentage of p53 mutations.

Urine cytology is very sensitive and specific for detecting CIS (95%).

Aggressive and high-risk: > 50% progress if untreated, ≤ 80% progression in G3 + CIS.

Primary CIS   isolated CIS with no history of bladder cancer, CIS or metachronous bladder cancer

Secondary CIS   detected on follow-up of a bladder cancer patient who did not have CIS before, often in association with high-grade disease

Concurrent CIS   in the presence of any urothelial tumour in urinary tract

SQUAMOUS CELL CARCINOMA

Rare in UK (4%) and often associated with chronic bladder irritation (e.g. long-term catheter, bladder stones, schistosomiasis).

Cystoscopy reveals ulcerated lesion on trigone or lateral walls.

ADENOCARCINOMA

Can be primary or secondary (distant metastasis or associated with urachal remnant).

Urachal remnant may present with visible haematuria and mucous discharge, histologically showing mucous-secreting cells and patient may be offered radical cystectomy + excision of urachus.

PRE-MALIGNANT LESIONS

The majority of bladder tumours are malignant, however there are pre-malignant lesions:

Keratinising squamous metaplasia
- seen in bladder exstrophy, schistosomiasis and chronic bladder inflammation

Urothelial dysplasia
- flat non-invasive lesion typified by nuclear clustering

Leucoplakia
- thick raised white plaques of squamous metaplasia on bladder surface, associated with recurrent UTIs, weak association with malignancy (similar to malakoplakia)

Cystitis cystica and non-keratinising squamous metaplasia are not pre-malignant.

INVESTIGATIONS

As per "Haematuria" station (history, examination, investigations, cystoscopy, proceed to TURBT)

For G1pTa TCC with no history of VH – upper tract imaging with CTU is not mandatory (risk of upper tract tumour is <1%)

TRANS-URETHRAL RESECTION OF BLADDER TUMOUR

The following response details in your viva the recommended steps for TURBT:
- Patient has provided full informed consent to procedure
- Fully prepped and draped with all elements of WHO checklist complete

- Perform bi-manual palpation under anaesthesia (if palpable suggests muscle-invasive)
- Full diagnostic cystoscopy with a continuous flow resectoscope
- Tumour resection with mono- or bi- polar diathermy loop, rollerball for haemostasis and fulguration of tumour edge to destroy any residual malignant tissue
- Biopsy of any other abnormal lesions searching for CIS / biopsy healthy mucosa in context of high-grade cytology and/or solid tumour / prostatic biopsies considered
- Bi-manual examination at the end (presence of mass strongly suggests T3 disease)
- Placement of a 3-way catheter and initiation of irrigation

Random biopsies for Ta / T1 disease rarely performed as chance of finding CIS is < 2%.

Obturator Kick

Tumours on the postero-lateral aspect of the bladder lie close to the obturator nerve which can be stimulated by the electric current and cause obturator kick / spasm.

The risk of this can be reduced by:
- keeping bladder under-filled during resection
- neuromuscular blockade (paralysis) under general anaesthesia
- reducing the voltage on the diathermy
- short, small controlled swipes using the loop

(direct obturator nerve block by lignocaine infiltration 2cm infero-lateral to pubic tubercle)

SECOND RESECTION

Recommendations for re-resection outlined in EAU guidelines [9] should be performed:
- incomplete initial TURBT
- no muscle in initial specimen (except TaLG / G1 and primary CIS)
- all T1 tumours (residual disease observed in 15–35% and upstaging noted in 30%

- all high-grade / G3 tumours (residual disease observed in 40% + upstaging in 23%)

Re-resection is critical for staging accuracy because the management of T1 disease differs significantly from T2.

Re-resection has been shown to increase recurrence-free survival rates.

NICE Guidelines recommend re-resection within 6 weeks of initial TURBT for all patients with high-risk NMIBC.

GRADING

In 2004 the International Society of Urological Pathology published a new histological classification of urothelial carcinoma compared to the older 1973 WHO classification. [10]

All grades 1 became PUNLMP or LG, all grades 2 became LG or HG, all grade 3 became HG.

The prognostic value of both systems have been demonstrated and neither are superior to the other and therefore both are used in current practice.

Table 5 – WHO vs. ISUP classification of urothelial carcinoma of the bladder

1973 WHO Grading	2004 ISUP Grading system (papillary lesions)
Grade 1: well-differentiated	Papillary urothelial neoplasm of low malignant potential (PUNLMP)
	Low-Grade papillary urothelial carcinoma
Grade 2: moderately differentiated	Low-Grade papillary urothelial carcinoma
	High-Grade papillary urothelial carcinoma
Grade 3: poorly differentiated	High-Grade papillary urothelial carcinoma

STAGING

Table 6 – TNM Classification for the staging of bladder cancer [9]

T – Primary tumour	
TX	Primary tumour cannot be assessed
T0	No evidence of primary tumour
Ta	Non-invasive papillary carcinoma
Tis	Carcinoma in situ: "flat tumour"
T1	Tumour invades sub-epithelial connective tissue
T2	Tumour invades muscle: • T2a – tumour invades superficial muscle (inner half) • T2b – tumour invades deep muscle (outer half)
T3	Tumour invades perivesical tissue: • T3a – microscopically • T3b – macroscopically (extravesical mass)
T4	Tumour invades other organs: • T4a – prostate, uterus or vagina • T4b – pelvic wall or abdominal wall
N – Lymph nodes	
NX	Regional lymph nodes cannot be assessed
N0	No regional lymph node metastasis
N1	Metastasis in single lymph node in the true pelvis (hypogastric, obturator, ext.iliac, presacral)
N2	Metastasis in multiple lymph nodes in true pelvis (hypogastric, obturator, ext.iliac, presacral)
N3	Metastasis in common iliac lymph node(s)
M – distant metastasis	
MX	Distant metastasis cannot be assessed
M0	No distant metastasis
M1	Distant metastasis: • M1a – non-regional lymph nodes • M1b – other distant metastasis

RISK STRATIFICATION

Table 7 – NICE bladder cancer: risk classification in non-muscle-invasive bladder cancer [11]

Low Risk	Solitary G1 / 2 (LG) pTa tumour < 3cm
	Any PUNLMP
Intermediate Risk	Solitary G1 / 2 (LG) pTa tumour > 3cm
	Multi-focal G1 / 2 (LG) pTa tumours
	HG G2 pTa tumour
	Any low-risk recurring NMIBC within 12 months
High Risk	G3 disease
	G2 / 3 pT1 tumour
	CIS
	Any aggressive variant

Table 8 – EAU (2018) risk group stratification [9]

Low Risk	Primary, solitary Ta, G1 (PUNLMP/LG), < 3cm, no CIS
Intermediate Risk	All tumours not defined in low- or high- risk groups
High Risk	T1 disease, G3 tumour, CIS
	Multiple + recurrent + large (> 3cm) Ta G1 / 2LG (all listed features present)
	Sub-group of highest risk: • G3pT1 (HG) + CIS • Multiple and/or large and/or recurrent G3pT1 disease

The EORTC and GUCG derived a scoring system from 7 trials in NMIBC.

The scores can be applied to the EORTC table to calculate percentage chance of progression and recurrence at 1 and 5 years.

These were derived from six most significant clinical and pathological factors found.

Table 9 – EORTC – GUCG scoring system [9]

Factor	Score	
	Recurrence	Progression
Number of tumours		
Single	0	0
2–7	3	3
≥ 8	6	3
Tumour size		
< 3 cm	0	0
≥ 3 cm	3	3
Prior recurrence rate		
Primary	0	0
≤ 1 per year	2	2
≤ 1 per year	4	2
T classification		
Ta	0	0
T1	1	4
Carcinoma in situ		
No	0	0
Yes	1	6
Grade		
G1	0	0
G2	1	0
G3	2	5
Total score	0–17	0–23

Table 10 – Probabilities of recurrence and progression (after 1 year and 5 years) (95% CI)

Recurrence score	% Probability recurrence at 1 year	% Probability recurrence at 5 years
0	15	31
1–4	24	46
5–9	38	62
10–17	61	78
Progression score		
0	0.2	0.8
2–6	1	6
7–13	5	17
14–23	17	45

Prior disease recurrence rate and number of tumours are the most important prognostic factors for disease recurrence.

Stage and grade are the most important factors for disease progression and disease-specific survival.

Age and grade are the most important factors for overall survival.

CIS will progress to invasive disease in over 50% if not treated.

Progression to muscle invasive disease will occur for patients in < 5 % of G1pTa, 10% multi-focal G1pT1, 30% G3pT1, 50% of CIS and 50–80% or G3 + CIS disease.

MANAGEMENT

MITOMYCIN-C

Administered as an intra-vesical chemotherapy agent (given 40mg in 40mL of saline over an hour).

MMC is an anti-tumour antibiotic causing DNA cross-linking in bladder tumour cells. [1] Systemic toxicity is rare however if irritative LUTS and genito-palmar rash occur then halt treatment.

Given as single instillation (SI) within hours (otherwise tumour cells implant and are covered by extra-cellular matrix) after TURBT to destroy circulating tumour cells and ablate residual tumour cells at resection site.

Sylvester et al. (2004) [12]

- published meta-analysis of 7 RCTs of TURBT + MMC vs. TURBT alone
- single MMC dose within 24 hours of TURBT: RR reduction of recurrence 39%, AR risk reduction of 12%
- NNT is 7 (to prevent a recurrence within 5 years)

i.e. reduces rate of recurrence but not progression

The most recent review suggested SI MMC only benefited those with EORTC score < 5 and recurrence rate of 1 or less per year.

For intermediate-risk patients, adjuvant MMC instillations may have an impact on recurrence, however there is no clear defined schedule for duration and frequency for this to be given.

HIVEC Trial, is currently comparing hyperthermia + MMC vs. MMC alone, in patients with intermediate risk disease.

BCG THERAPY

Bacillus Calmette-Guerin (live attenuated mycobacterium bovis)

Available strains include Connaught, OncoTice and RIVM with comparable efficacies.

Mechanism of action poorly understood – attaches to urothelium via fibronectin receptor, internalised within the cell, acting as immune stimulant by up-regulating cytokine production (IL-6 and IL-8) within bladder wall and mediating macrophage chemotaxis.

Administered via catheter which is removed, patient asked to retain for 2 hours and then void whilst sitting down to avoid contamination and wash hands with bleach.

Indications

Comparable efficacy with MMC for low- and intermediate- risk groups and therefore not recommended first line due to added toxicity risk.

In high-risk superficial disease it is recommended.

Meta-analysis by Sylvester et al. (2002) of 24 trials and 4800 patients found 27% RR reduction (4% ARR) progression to muscle-invasive disease with maintenance BCG, 2.5 year follow up. [13]

Maintenance BCG only (i.e. not induction BCG) will reduce the risk of disease progression in both papillary and CIS tumours.

The full maintenance protocol involves 27 instillations over 3 years (Lamm's regime).

BCG can also be given 2nd line for patients with NMIBC recurrence after MMC regimen.

Contraindications

- immuno-suppressed patients
- pregnant or breast-feeding women
- known haematological malignancy
- active TB
- recent traumatic catheterisation (concern of systemic absorption)
- active heavy haematuria on the day of planned treatment
- active urinary tract infection
- prior TURBT within < 2 weeks
- cirrhosis or liver disease (isoniazid cannot be given if patients develop BCG-sepsis
- total incontinence (patient cannot retain BCG)

Risks and Toxicity

Cystitis symptoms are the most common side-effect of BCG treatment.

Low-grade fever and myalgia are also common and self-limiting symptoms.

BCG sepsis must be considered if patient on BCG therapy experiences fever / malaise / headaches:

- admit as emergency
- systematic A-E resuscitation and sepsis-6 bundle
- start treatment with anti-tuberculous therapy
- liaise with microbiology and respiratory medicine

Lower-dose BCG therapy has been considered (CUETO study looked at 1/3 dose vs. full dose) however toxicities were comparable whilst possible higher recurrence rate for lower dose.

BCG Failure

Patients with a low-grade recurrence after BCG do not constitute BCG failure.

High-grade recurrences after BCG imply that patient is unlikely to respond to further BCG, and radical cystectomy is the treatment of choice (further BCG remains an option (NICE 2020)).

Prompt re-discussion at the cancer MDT is recommended.

Interferon-alpha, can be used as 50 mega-units + 1/3 BCG dose for patients who fail BCG therapy and shows increased response rate of 50%.

BCG Schedule

The optimal number of induction instillations, frequency and duration of maintenance instillations is not currently defined.

The EORTC showed that 3-year maintenance reduced recurrence rate when compared to 1-year maintenance for high-risk disease only (not intermediate).

An example includes Lamm's regime:
- post-TURBT BCG weekly for 6 weeks
- at 3 months, weekly for 3 weeks
- at 6 months, weekly for 3 weeks
- every 6 months thereafter, weekly for 3 weeks, until 3 years

During treatment you should avoid quinolone therapy as this can affect efficacy.

RE-RESECTION

NICE Guidelines recommends re-resection for newly diagnosed NMIBC high-risk group (Table 11).

Re-resection should be offered < 6 weeks from histological diagnosis.

This is because studies have shown that residual disease after TURBT is found in 33–55% of T1 tumours, and disease upstaging may occur in ≤ 30% after re-resection. [1]

Staging accuracy is paramount as management of T1 vs. T2 disease differs significantly.

RADICAL CYSTECTOMY

Covered in the "MIBC" station.

G3PT1 DISEASE MANAGEMENT

1/3 of patients will never have recurrence, 1/3 will die of metastatic disease and 1/3 will undergo deferred radical cystectomy (RC).

Aggressive management is warranted due to the high risk of disease progression.

- Re-resection within 6 weeks [NICE] – due to 23% risk of upstaging
- Discuss at uro-oncology MDT – consider adjuvant BCG vs. primary RC
- If BCG fails, then consider RC

CIS MANAGEMENT

CIS treatment, mainstay is maintenance 3 years intra-vesical BCG, with half of patients disease-free at 5 years and 1/3 at 10 years.

Overall initial complete response is 75% and an important prognostic indicator – 1/10 patients who respond will progress to muscle-invasive disease, compared to 2/3 of non-responders.

Sylvester et al. meta-analysis suggested that BCG is superior to MMC for treating CIS.

RECURRENT NMIBC (LOW RISK)

Consider fulguration without biopsy for patients with recurrent NMIBC provided: [11]

- previous NMIBC was low-risk
- disease-free interval of ≥ 6 months
- solitary papillary recurrence
- tumour diameter ≤ 3mm

NICE (2020) MANAGEMENT SUMMARY

Table 11 – NICE 2020 management options per risk stratification group

RISK GROUP	INVESTIGATION	TREATMENT	FOLLOW-UP
Low	Cystoscopy Cytology Histopathology	SI MMC	Cystoscopy 3 & 12 months If no recurrence, discharge at 12 months
Intermediate	Cystoscopy Cytology Histopathology	SI MMC x6 maintenance MMC	Cystoscopy 3, 9 & 18 months Yearly thereafter Discharge after 5 years disease-free
High	Cystoscopy Cytology Histopathology	SI MMC Re-resection < 6 weeks BCG vs RC	Cystoscopy 3 monthly for 2 years Cystoscopy 6 monthly for 2 years Lifelong yearly cystoscopy thereafter

MUSCLE-INVASIVE BLADDER CANCER

OVERVIEW

Primary presentation of MIBC will feature in 25% of new bladder cancer patients.

For the 75% presenting with superficial disease, approximately a quarter will progress to muscle-invasive disease.

All MIBC cases are by definition high-grade urothelial carcinomas, and therefore grading MIBC does not provide prognostic value.

ASSESSMENT

Symptoms

Painless visible haematuria is the most common presenting symptom.

Pelvic pain, urinary tract obstruction and fistulation are all symptoms of advanced disease.

Examination

Bi-manual (rectal – vaginal) palpation in the presence of a chaperone should be undertaken to identify a palpable mass or mass fixed to the pelvic wall.

Cystoscopy

There is currently no role for photodynamic diagnosis (PDD) in the standard diagnosis of MIBC, although it can be used to detect CIS in the context of T1 disease.

Re-Resection

Recall that 1/3 to 1/2 of high-grade NMIBC will harbour residual disease after initial resection, which will result in being upstaged after re-resection is performed.

MUSCLE-INVASIVE BLADDER CANCER

Concomitant Prostate Cancer

Prostate cancer is found in 25–40 % of cysto-prostatectomy specimens, therefore recommended patient undergoes PSA monitoring as part of their follow-up plan.

Impact on overall survival of this is not known.

IMAGING

CT SCAN

NICE Guidelines and EAU recommend CT TAP with urographic phase for correct staging of MIBC.

CT has similar accuracy to MRI for local staging and in detecting extra-vesical disease extension (i.e. differentiating T2 from T3b disease) or local organs.

CT is inferior to MRI in determining depth of bladder wall involvement as it cannot discern the different wall layers (i.e. cannot differentiate between Ta to T3a tumours).

CT and MRI are comparable for lymph node assessment – equivocal cases can be further evaluated with PET-CT scan [NICE Guideline].

MRI SCAN

Can be used as an alternative to CT scan for local staging and metastatic disease assessment within the abdomen.

MRI has better soft-tissue resolution and can distinguish invasion of different bladder wall layers.

MRI should not be used if eGFR < 30 ml / min.

Lymph Node Imaging

Assessment of LNs based solely on size is a limitation as both CT and MRI are unable to identify metastases in normal-size or slightly enlarged LNs.

Pelvic nodes > 8mm and abdominal nodes > 10mm are taken as significant.

Sensitivity and specificity of the imaging techniques is low.

PROGNOSTIC EVALUATION

Tumour and nodal staging are the main prognostic factors in the radical treatment of MIBC.

Insufficient evidence exists to recommend p53 as prognostic marker in high-risk MIBC.

All factors that will predispose a patient to a poorer outcome from surgery (poor fitness, extremes of BMI, low albumin) are also relevant.

Evaluation of comorbidity is preferable as an indicator for life expectancy rather than patient age.

Charlson Comorbidity Index

The CCI is a score ranging from 0–30, calculated by healthcare professionals depending on comorbidities of the patient (Table 12).

This index has been shown to be an independent prognostic factor for peri-operative mortality and 5-year all-cause mortality after radical cystectomy. [14]

Risk categories by score points include low (0), medium (1–3) and high (≥4). [15]

Alternative comorbidity indices include Elixhauser index and ECOG performances status.

EAU Guidelines (2019) recommend against using ASA score for basing decision for radical cystectomy, but rather a validated score such as CCI. [16]

Table 12 – Charlson Comorbidity Index [16]

Score	Condition
1	50–60 years, IHD, heart failure, COPD, PVD, dementia, diabetes, stroke, mild liver disease, peptic ulcer disease
2	61–70 years, Localised tumour, leukaemia, lymphoma, moderate / end stage renal failure
3	71–80 years, Moderate / severe liver disease
4	81–90 years
5	> 90 years
6	Metastatic solid tumour, AIDS

WHO Performance Status

Performance status is a score that estimates the ability of the patient to perform certain activities of daily living without assistance from others.

Important factor for determining suitability of treatment as well as for selection criteria for clinical trials.

Table 13 – WHO (and ECOG) Performance status [17]

Performance Status	Description
0	able to carry out all normal activity without restriction
1	restricted in strenuous activity but ambulatory and able to carry out light work
2	ambulatory and capable of all self-care but unable to carry out any work activities; up and about more than 50% of waking hours
3	symptomatic and in a chair or in bed for greater than 50% of the day but not bedridden
4	completely disabled; cannot carry out any self-care; totally confined to bed or chair.

Cardio-Pulmonary Exercise Test (CPEX or CPET)

CPEX carried out as outpatient procedure. Patient sits on bicycle/walks on treadmill and is connected to a 12 lead ECG, blood pressure cuff and pulse oximeter.

Three ventilatory variables are measured:
- oxygen consumption
- carbon dioxide excretion
- minute ventilation

The exercise resistance is gradually increased over 10–15 minutes.

CPEX is a functional assessment of cardiopulmonary reserve and is becoming routine in the preoperative assessment of patients undergoing major surgery (e.g. cystectomy).

Anaerobic threshold is the point at which aerobic metabolism is no longer adequate and anaerobic supplementation begins (note that aerobic respiration does not cease).

- CPEX can also measure this by different signatures on gas exchange
- The cut off for major surgery: anaerobic threshold ≥ 11mL / kg / minute [18]

TREATMENT

TREATMENT FAILURE OF NMIBC

According to EAU Guidelines it is reasonable to propose immediate RC to patients with NMIBC who are at the highest risk of progression:

- T1 tumours
- G3 (HG) and/or CIS (even higher if multiple, recurrent, within prostatic urethra)
- multiple and recurrent and large (>3cm) G1G2 pTa tumours (all conditions met)
- unusual histology, lympho-vascular invasion
- BCG-failures: recurrent CIS or high-grade, MIBC on surveillance cystoscopy

NEO-ADJUVANT CHEMOTHERAPY

NC administered prior to radical surgery has evidence of benefit obtained from meta-analysis "Advanced Bladder Cancer (ABC)" (2005) of 5% absolute improvement in 5-year survival. [19]

NICE 2020 recommends using cisplatin combination regimen before offering RC or EBRT to patients with newly diagnosed MIBC, for those for whom such a regimen is suitable. [20]

EAU 2019 recommends NC should be offered for T2 – T4a disease (i.e. not in RC for NMIBC). [16]

Combination regimens includes GC (gemcitabine + cisplatin) or MVAC (methotrexate, vinblastine, Adriamycin, cisplatin).

Ensure the patient has an opportunity to discuss the risks and benefits of NC with an oncologist.

Considerations regarding NC include:
- delivery at earliest time-point (lowest burden of micro-metastatic disease)
- tolerability of chemotherapy better before major surgery

- NC does not affect outcome of surgical morbidity
- patients have to be fit for cisplatin-combination therapy

ADJUVANT CHEMOTHERAPY

There is currently no evidence to support routinely giving adjuvant chemotherapy to patients who have undergone radical surgery.

NICE (2020) recommends considering adjuvant cisplatin combination chemotherapy after RC for patients whose RC histology showed MIBC and / or LN positive disease, but that did not receive NC prior to RC as their pre-RC histology was NMIBC. [20]

RADICAL EXTERNAL BEAM RADIOTHERAPY (EBRT)

Alternative to major surgery for those unfit or unwilling to have RC.

There are no RCTs comparing the two modalities to date, however 5-year survival rates reportedly better in RC (this could be as the EBRT patients were less fit to begin with).

Typical dose is 66 Gy over 6 weeks. Target field is bladder only.

There is no benefit to survival in giving neo-adjuvant EBRT prior to RC.

CIS, SCC and adenocarcinoma are poorly sensitive to EBRT.

NC is beneficial for patients undergoing EBRT and should be offered.

EBRT should not be considered in patients with severe irritative LUTS, previous pelvic irradiation, inflammatory bowel disease and upper tract obstruction.

Salvage cystectomy is an option in select cases with 5-year survival rates < 50%.

Follow-up After EBRT

After EBRT consider a follow-up protocol comprising of: [20]
- rigid cystoscopy (3 months)
- flexible cystoscopy (6 months and then 3 monthly for 2 years and then 6 monthly for 2 years)
- imaging for upper tract monitoring (annual)
- imaging for local / distant recurrence using CT TAP (6, 12 and 24 months)

RADICAL CYSTECTOMY (RC)

The most effective treatment for localised MIBC.

Indicated for muscle-invasive TCC, SCC, adenocarcinoma, G3T1 + CIS, BCG-failures, obstructed upper-tracts, high-volume recurrent papillary disease, select cases of EBRT failure.

Timing & Delay of RC

Delays of > 12 weeks should be avoided as this has a negative impact on outcome.

This is relevant when considering the timely delivery of NC.

Standard RC Technique

Midline incision trans-peritoneal or extra-peritoneal approach.

Remove entire bladder & peri-vesical fat, prostate, seminal vesicles, distal ureters, regional lymph node dissection, uterus & anterior vaginal wall & entire urethra in women.

Divide ureters close to bladder and anastomose to chosen technique of urinary diversion, protect these with ureteric stents.

Lymph Node Dissection

LND has important clinical significance in RC related to the two main aspects of nodal dissection: therapeutic vs. staging instrument.

LN involvement is a strong predictor of 5-year CSS: N- 80% and N+ 40%.

There is currently no consensus on the extent of LND that should be undertaken in RC: [16]

- *standard*, up to common iliac bifurcation (internal iliac, pre-sacral, external iliac LN)
- *extended*, includes standard + LN up to aortic bifurcation
- *super-extended*, dissection reaches the inferior mesenteric artery level cranially

Overall suggested that >10 LN should be dissected (adequate for staging) and an increasing number of dissected LN correlates with overall survival and progression-free survival.

Primary Urethrectomy

Recommended to preserve the urethra if frozen section margins are negative (positive margin is an absolute contra-indication to neobladder formation).

Primary urethrectomy is advised if urethral margins are positive, primary tumour at bladder neck or within prostatic urethra, or with extensive CIS disease.

Risk of urethral recurrence is lower with the use of neobladder (4%) vs. ileal conduit (8%) (suggesting that urine is protective in this setting).

The risk of urethral recurrence rises to ≤ 18% in presence of prostatic urethral involvement.

Sexual Preserving Techniques

Different approaches for preserving sexual function in men have been described, concern remains regarding their oncological outcome, and no approach has been shown to be superior.

The preserving techniques should not be offered routinely but only for strongly motivated patients and their MIBC must be localised, not invading the prostate or bladder neck.

Prostate sparing, including vas, seminal vesicles and NVBs

Capsule sparing, as for prostate-sparing but prostate adenoma is removed.

Seminal sparing, preserving seminal vesicles, vas, NVBs

Nerve sparing, the NVBs are the only tissue left in place.

Open vs. Lap vs. Robot-Assisted RC

There is no clear evidence to date to support a superior oncological outcome with any operative modality of RC (open vs. robotic vs. laparoscopic).

Robotic-assisted has shorter hospital stay, longer operative time, increased costs, lower complication rates and less blood-loss when compared to open cystectomy.

Surgeon experience and institutional volume are considered the key factors for outcome for both open and robot-assisted, rather than the technique itself.

Quality of Life (QoL) outcomes appear to be comparable long-term.

STATION 1: UROLOGICAL ONCOLOGY 1

Follow-up After RC

After RC consider a follow-up protocol comprising of: [20]

- imaging for upper tract monitoring for hydronephrosis / stones / cancer (annual), and
- imaging for local / distant recurrence using CT TAP (6, 12 and 24 months), and
- blood tests for metabolic acidosis, B12 and folate deficiency (annual)
- urethroscopy and / or urethral washing cytology in defunctioned urethras (annual for 5 years)

Palliative Cystectomy

Patients with locally advanced tumours (e.g. T4b) may experience debilitating symptoms such as intractable haematuria, pain and urinary obstruction.

Palliative cystectomy with urinary diversion is feasible but carries the greatest morbidity, EAU 2019 recommends alternatives such as RTx or nephrostomy tube insertion if at all possible. [16]

COMPLICATIONS AFTER RC

RC is associated with mortality of 3% and morbidity of 30%.

Table 14 – Risks and complications after RC

	Immediate	Early	Late
Risks of RC	• intra-operative death • Bleeding / transfusion	• DVT / PE • Infection: chest, wound • Ileo-ileal anastomotic leak • Uretero-ileal leak • Stroke, MI, death	• Incisional/para-stomal hernias • Stomal stenosis • Anastomotic stricture • Hyperchloraemic metabolic acidosis • Cancer recurrence • Vaginal shortening

In addition, patients undergoing ortho-topic neo-bladder formation should be informed of the risks of erectile dysfunction, loss of ejaculation and retention of urine.

During the FRCS(Urol) viva, make sure complications are discussed with reference to the Clavien-Dindo classification of surgical complications. (Table 15)

Table 15 – Clavien-Dindo classification of surgical complications

Clavien-Dindo Grade	Nature of complication
1	Deviation from normal post-operative course without need for pharmacological / surgical / endoscopic / radiological treatment (i.e. anti-emetic / pyretic, analgesics or bedside wound opening are acceptable)
2	Requiring pharmacological treatment with drugs other than allowed for Grade 1 (e.g. blood transfusion, antibiotics, TPN)
3	Requiring surgical / endoscopic / radiological intervention: 3a – under regional / local anaesthesia 3b – under GA
4	Life-threatening complication requiring ITU: 4a – single-organ dysfunction 4b – multi-organ dysfunction
5	Patient death

Hyperchloraemic Metabolic Acidosis

Very common after ileal conduit formation, in most cases sub-clinical and in small proportion of patients it is observed long-term.

Bowel secretes (sodium in exchange of hydrogen) and (bicarbonate in exchange of chloride).

Bowel exposed to urine re-absorbs acid & chloride leading to chronic acid load (hyperchloraemic metabolic acidosis) made worse by lower baseline kidney function and the use of colonic instead of ileal segments.

This can be treated with oral sodium bicarbonate, although use limited by flatulence.

Other Metabolic Abnormalities

Low Potassium, intestinal secretory loss and renal wasting. Hypokalaemia can be further worsened in the process of correcting the metabolic acidosis.

Low calcium, renal wasting and depletion of body calcium stores (the chronic metabolic acidosis is buffered by bone carbonate) and patient may require calcium supplementation.

Low magnesium.

Macrocytic anaemia, as vitamin B12 absorption occurs in terminal ileum (vit. B12 stores are sufficient for 3 years so deficiency may not become apparent until this time).

Bone De-mineralisation

Mobilisation of calcium and carbonate from bones to buffer the chronic metabolic acidosis can lead to osteomalacia.

Furthermore acidosis impairs renal activation of vitamin-D, which is essential for bone mineralisation, and activates osteoclast activity.

URINARY DIVERSION

NICE (2020) recommends offering continent urinary diversion in RC if no strong contraindications such as cognitive impairment, impaired renal function or significant bowel disease. [20]

Anatomically, there are three alternatives used for diversion after cystectomy:

- abdominal e.g. ileal or colonic conduit
- urethral, various forms of gastro-intestinal pouches attached to urethra (e.g. neobladder)
- rectosigmoid diversions

Ileal Conduit

The most common method of urinary diversion in the UK is the ileal conduit (15cm).

Early complications – ileum / obstruction, anastomotic leak, stenosis, conduit ischaemia

Late complications – stomal stenosis, para-stomal herniation

Metabolic acidosis is less common with ileal conduit when compared to neobladder.

Bricker technique – anastomosis by spatulating and anastomosing each ureter to the serosa of the bowel separately

Wallace 1 technique – both ureters spatulated to same length, medial walls anastomosed together and free edges of conjoined ureters are anastomosed to proximal end of open bowel segment.

Orthotopic Neobladder

The terminal ileum is the gastro-intestinal segment of choice for bladder substitution, however a greater length (60cm) is required thus increasing the risk of metabolic sequelae.

Emptying of the reservoir requires abdominal straining, intestinal peristalsis, sphincter relaxation.

90% are continent by day (slightly less by night).

Age > 80 years is the threshold above which orthotopic neobladder is not recommended.

The Studer neobladder is a commonly used technique in the UK.

Uretero-colonic Diversion

Most indications for this procedure have become obsolete due to the risk of upper tract infections and increased risk of colonic malignancy ($\leq$ 29% risk at 20 years follow up).

Gas may be seen in the upper tracts on imaging due to reflux.

Pre-operatively the "porridge test" to assess suitability for uretero-colonic diversion involves flushing 500mL of liquid per rectum and asking patient to hold this in situ for $\geq$ 1 hour.

Avoids the use of stoma bag in countries where stoma care or community costs cannot be met.

Uretero-cutaneostomy

This is the simplest form of cutaneous diversion, reducing operative time, post-operative support and length of hospital stay when compared to ileal conduit.

Option for elderly and otherwise compromised patients.

EBRT VS. RC

Table 16 – risks and benefits for RC vs. EBRT as radical treatment for MIBC

	EBRT	RC
Benefits	Avoids major surgery	Full staging available
	Preserves bladder	Better 5-year survival rates?
		Can treat CIS
Risks	LUTS,	Bleeding
	Small bladder capacity,	Infection
	Proctitis	DVT / PE
	Second malignancy	Collection / anastomotic leak
		Stomal stenosis
		Hyperchloraemic metabolic acidosis

PARTIAL CYSTECTOMY (PC)

Approximately 10% of patients with bladder cancer are candidates for PC.

Laparoscopic PC is not routine and 5-year survival after open surgery is 50%.

Suitable for those with small lesions and a lack of concurrent CIS (e.g. 1cm T2 lesion on the dome), tumour in diverticulum.

Multiple tumours, CIS, tumours close to ureteric orifices or on trigone are not suitable for PC.

METASTATIC DISEASE

10% of patients with bladder cancer present with metastases at diagnosis.

50% of patients undergoing RC for MIBC will relapse, prognosis is in the order of months.

Performance status, presence of visceral metastases and low Hb are prognostic factors relevant in metastatic bladder cancer.

MANAGEMENT

- Thorough assessment
- Debulking TURBT – to obtain histology and reduce haematuria and voiding symptoms
- MDT Discussion
- Palliative chemotherapy – providing adequate performance status and renal function

CHEMOTHERAPY

TCC is a chemo-sensitive cancer.

Combination (cisplatin-based) therapy is more effective than single-agent use.

MVAC is a standard combination and can achieve median survival of 14 months, assess Karnovsky status prior to offering this as an option.

URACHAL TUMOUR

Very rare, usually adenocarcinoma (85%) but can also be SCCa or TCC, located at bladder dome.

Treatment is partial cystectomy or RC, 5-year survival ~ 50%.

Bladder adenocarcinomas are more common in females, however urachal tumours are more common in men.

RENAL CANCER

EPIDEMIOLOGY

3% of all cancers

Peak incidence 60–70 years of age

Male to female is 1.5 : 1.

Clear-cell RCC 80%, papillary RCC 15%, chromophobe RCC 5%

Leiomyosarcoma is the most common type of renal sarcoma.

RISK FACTORS

Smoking, obesity, hypertension, 1st degree affected relative

Patients on dialysis (with their native kidneys in situ) – 3–6x risk

Hereditary	(5–8%) VHL syndrome, hereditary papillary renal cell carcinoma (HPRC), hereditary leiomyomatosis and papillary RCC (HLRCC), Birt-Hogg-Dube' syndrome
Anatomical	polycystic kidney disease, horse-shoe kidney
Occupational	asbestos, cadmium

HEREDITARY CONDITIONS

Von-Hippel Lindau Disease

Autosomal dominant (chromosome 3) genetic disorder affecting males and females equally

Affecting 1 / 36,000 live births [21]

VHL occurs due to loss of both copies of tumour suppressor gene at chromosome 3 (3p25–26), which results in dysregulation of hypoxia inducible factors (HIF) 1 & 2.

As such, cells lacking VHL gene in hypoxic conditions will accumulate HIF-1. This will over-express genes related to angiogenesis (VEGF and PDGF) and cell-division.

Up-regulation of VEGF is the most prominent angiogenic factor in RCC.

VHL characterised by phaeochromocytoma, visceral / pancreatic cysts and neuro-endocrine tumours, cerebellar haemangioblastoma and RCCs (often multi-focal).

Most tumours in VHL share the characteristic of hyper-vascularity.

Loss of vision is common due to angiomatosis (nests of proliferating capillaries) in the retina.

RCC and cysts typically evolve in multiple sites in the kidney after 20 years of age (> 3cm in size is thought to be high-risk for malignant transformation.

Treatment should focus on aim of maintaining nephrons. Monitor with US first and then regular surveillance CT / MRI once lesions larger (> 2 cm), consider ablative therapies or PN for smaller lesions.

Ultimately patient may require renal replacement therapy, role of transplantation is limited.

Main causes of death are related to RCC and haemangioblastoma complications. [21]

Birt-Hogg-Dube' Syndrome

Autosomal dominant genetic condition that can cause susceptibility to kidney cancer, renal and pulmonary cysts, benign tumours of hair follicles (fibrofolliculomas)

BHD arises from mutations of the FLCN gene on chromosome 17p. [22]

Fibrofolliculomas are mainly in the facial region and are the most common manifestation of BHD; pulmonary cysts may lead to spontaneous pneumothorax.

The most common renal tumour in BHD is mixed oncocytoma and chromophobe.

Hereditary Papillary Renal Cell Carcinoma (type 1 papillary)

HPRC follows autosomal dominant inheritance, in familial cases is associated with mutation of *met* oncogene on chromosome 7.

Increases risk of type 1 papillary RCC (multiple / bilateral).

Unlike VHL for example, it does not increase risk of tumours elsewhere. [23]

Hereditary Leiomyomatosis and Renal Cell Carcinoma (Type 2 Papillary) (or Reed's Syndrome)

Autosomal dominant genetic condition.

Arises due to mutations of the fumarate hydratase gene (works in the Kreb's cycle).

HLRCC is the most aggressive form of hereditary RCC condition and tends to have an earlier age of onset and higher grade cancers than HPRC.

Non-oncological manifestations include uterine fibroids and cutaneous leiomyomas. [23]

ANGIOMYOLIPOMA

Benign mesenchymal tumour composed of peri-vascular epithelioid cells containing blood vessels, immature smooth muscle and fat.

Female to male is 4 : 1, more common on the right side (80%), commonly present as bilateral / multifocal tumours (80%), mean age at presentation 30 years.

20% are due to tuberous sclerosis (autosomal dominant condition characterised by mental retardation and epilepsy). [24]

They have a steady growth rate of 20% per year (5% / year if sporadic).

The main risk they pose is acute bleeding into retroperitoneum or collecting system.

Imaging

More than half are incidentally diagnosed on routine imaging, otherwise after investigations for flank pain, visible haematuria or palpable mass. [24]

USS shows echo-bright pattern as fat reflects US waves and there is no acoustic shadow (distinguishing it from calculus). CT has low Hounsfield units (< 10).

Treatment

Active surveillance (AS) is considered first line option for most AMLs.

4cm is considered cut-off for AS. [25]

Factors that should urge toward treating AML include:
- > 4cm size and/or symptomatic AMLs
- pregnant women (pose higher risk of bleeding)
- lipid-poor AML (pose higher risk of bleeding)

Treatment includes selective arterial embolization (1st line) or cryotherapy or RFA, or indeed partial / simple nephrectomy.

AML volume (e.g. multiple AML) can be reduced prior to surgical intervention by the MTOR inhibitor everolimus [EAU Guidelines].

Tuberous Sclerosis

Autosomal dominant condition, mapped to TSC1 (chromosome 9, coding for hamartin) and TSC2 (chromosome 16, coding for tuberin). [26]

Features the following manifestations:
- hamartomas in the central nervous system (epilepsy, learning difficulty)
- AML in kidneys and renal cysts
- skin / facial angiofibromas
- rhabdomyomas in the heart

Wunderlich Syndrome

Rare condition of spontaneous acute renal haemorrhage into retro-peritoneal space. [27]

Presents with "Lenk's triad": flank pain, palpable mass and hypovolaemic shock.

AMLs are the most common cause of Wunderlich syndrome. Other causes include malignant neoplasm, rupture of renal artery aneurysm, anti-coagulant therapy.

Wunderlich syndrome can be treated conservatively if the patient is haemodynamically stable, otherwise emergency embolization or nephrectomy may be required.

DIAGNOSIS

PRESENTATION

50% of RCCs are incidentally diagnosed on routine imaging.

For the symptomatic RCCs, the most common presenting symptom is visible haematuria.

The classic triad of "loin pain, visible haematuria and palpable mass" is uncommon (< 10%) and correlates with aggressive histology and advanced disease.

Symptoms of para-neoplastic manifestations occur in 30% (Table 17).

Table 17 – Para-neoplastic symptoms associated with RCC

Symptom	Aetiology
Hypertension	renin production by the primary tumour (acting on the renin angiotensin aldosterone system)
Polycythaemia	over-production of EPO
Hypercalcaemia	non-metastatic – parathyroid hormone-like peptide produced by RCC cells, metastatic – osteolytic breakdown
Stauffer's syndrome	signs / symptoms of liver abnormalities in absence of liver metastases e.g. raised LFTs, fever, weight-loss, thrombocytopenia (IL-6 production)

IMAGING

CT UROGRAM

Phase 1 – non-contrast, visualisation of calcifications/stones/fat as well as providing baseline attenuation (Hounsfield) for assessing enhancement post-contrast

Phase 2 – nephrographic, (100 sec. post-contrast) highest sensitivity in detecting renal masses and comparison with unenhanced images is paramount to seek enhancement

Phase 3 – excretory, (10 minutes post-contrast) opacification of collecting systems, ureters and bladder, allowing evaluation of urothelium

CT urogram utilises an iodine-based contrast medium

If the results of CT-urogram are inconclusive, contrast-enhanced ultrasound is a valuable alternative to further characterise renal lesions.

Split-bolus technique can be used to reduce radiation dose (protocols vary):
- 75mL (IV) contrast at start
- wait for 5–8 minutes
- further 75mL (IV) contrast
- start scanning after ~ 60 seconds

Aims to put together in a single image acquisition both the nephrographic and excretory phases, thus reducing the radiation dose to the patient. [28]

CT thorax should be undertaken simultaneously for evaluation of metastases.

Enhancement

The most important criterion for differentiating malignant lesions from benign.

Suggests the presence of vascular tissue or communication with the collecting system.

A *change of > 15 Hounsfield units* between pre- and post- contrast images is considered significant in pointing toward a malignant diagnosis. [29]

MR-UROGRAM

Indicated in patients who are allergic to IV contrast medium, are pregnant or in renal failure.

Option for patients with hereditary conditions for surveillance concerned radiation exposure.

BOSNIAK CLASSIFICATION OF RENAL CYSTS

Classification based on CT used to determine follow-up and predict risk of underlying malignancy:

Type 1 – benign and can be discharged.

Type 2 – follow-up to look for change in size / new features (10% risk of transformation).

Type 3 – almost half will be malignant – surgery should be considered.

Type 4 – > 90% of these cysts will be malignant and nephrectomy should be considered.

Table 18 – Description and management of Bosniak cysts

Bosniak Type	Features	Follow-up
I	Simple benign cyst, hairline-thin wall. No separations, calcification, solid components. Non-enhancing. Same density as water	Benign
II	May contain a few hairline septa. Fine calcification may be present in wall or septa. Non-enhancing. Uniformly high attenuation < 3cm in size	Benign
IIF	More hairline-thin septa (with minimal enhancement). Minimal thickening of septa or wall. May contain calcification (no enhancement). No enhancing soft-tissue elements. High attenuation renal lesions > 3 cm	Follow-up (Some are malignant)
III	Indeterminate cystic masses. Thickened irregular walls or septa (enhancing)	Surgery or Surveillance (50% are malignant)
IV	Enhancing soft-tissue components	Surgery (Most are malignant)

RENAL TUMOUR BIOPSY

RTB via US- or CT- guided means has gained popularity due to increasing number of small indeterminate masses being diagnosed incidentally.

Indications for RTB include:

- uncertainty regarding nature of the lesion (e.g. lipid-poor AML) (patient for active treatment)
- prior to systemic therapy (i.e. metastatic RCC)

- prior to cryotherapy or RFA
- prior to tumour surveillance

For frail / co-morbid patients unfit for intervention, RTB is not indicated.

A clearly enhancing lesion already listed for surgery does not require a prior biopsy.

Sensitivity, specificity and diagnostic accuracy are high. Marconi et al. (2016) systematic review of > 50 studies and > 5000 patients undergoing RTB: [30]

- 92% median diagnostic rate
- Sensitivity / specificity > 99%

Risk of seeding is a historical concern and extremely low.

For large tumour, avoid sampling central area which may be necrotic.

STAGING

Table 19 – TNM classification for staging of renal cell carcinoma [31]

T – Primary Tumour	
TX	Primary tumour cannot be assessed
T0	No evidence of primary tumour
T1	Tumour ≤ 7cm in greatest dimension, limited to the kidney • T1a – tumour ≤ 4cm • T1b – tumour > 4cm but ≤ 7cm
T2	Tumour > 7cm in greatest dimension, limited to the kidney • T2a – tumour > 7cm but ≤ 10cm • T2b – tumour > 10cm, limited to the kidney
T3	Tumour extends into major veins or perinephric tissues, but not into ipsilateral adrenal gland and not beyond Gerota's fascia • T3a – extends into renal vein or segmental branches or tumour invades perirenal / sinus fat but not beyond Gerota's fascia • T3b – tumour grossly extends into the IVC below the diaphragm • T3c – tumour grossly extends into the IVC above the diaphragm or invades IVC wall
T4	Tumour invades beyond Gerota's fascia (including into ipsilateral adrenal gland)

N – Lymph nodes	
NX	Regional lymph nodes cannot be assessed
N0	No regional lymph node metastasis
N1	Metastasis in regional lymph node(s)
M – Metastasis	
M0	No distant metastasis
M1	Distant metastasis (includes contralateral adrenal gland involvement)

Staging of IVC Involvement

RCC are accompanied by IVC involvement in ≤ 10% of cases, with surgical resection being the only curative option available. [32]

The different stages of IVC involvement of renal tumour is shown in (Image 1). [33]

- Level I – tumour thrombus extending to renal vein and < 2cm above renal vein orifice
- Level II – tumour thrombus extending > 2cm above renal vein orifice but below hepatic veins
- Level III – tumour thrombus extending above hepatic veins but below the diaphragm
- Level IV – tumour thrombus extending above the diaphragm

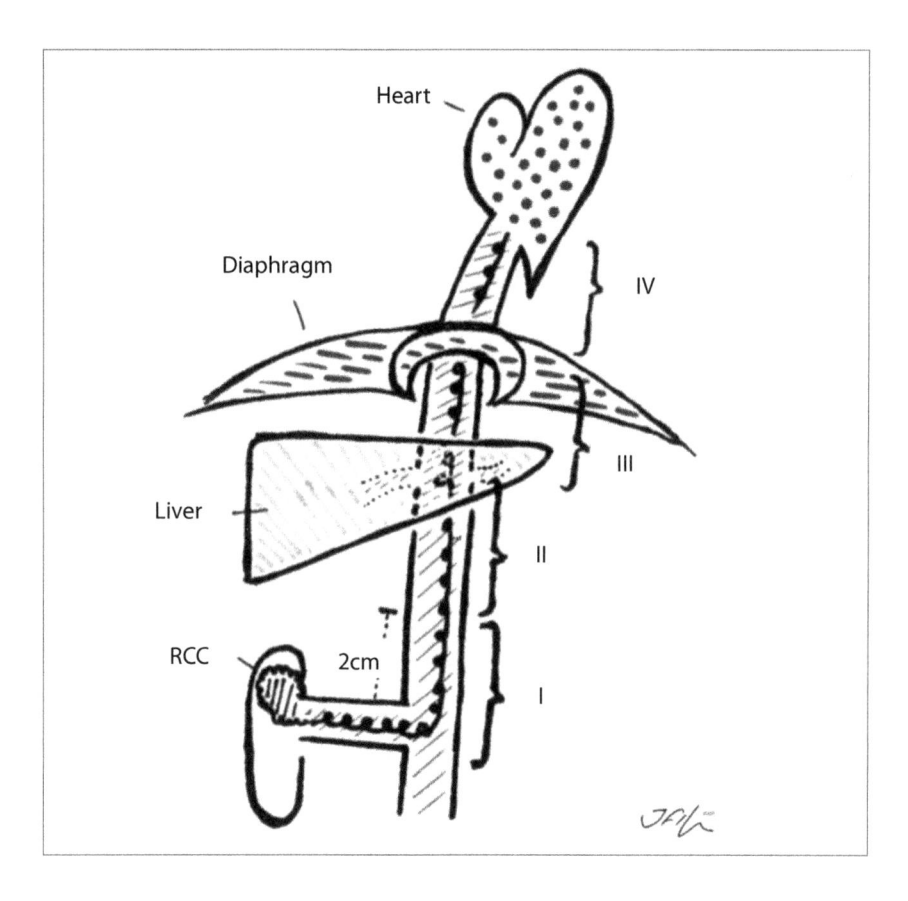

Image 1 –Stages of IVC involvement of renal tumour

PROGNOSTIC FACTORS

Anatomical factors (as per TNM staging), histology and clinical factors (e.g. performance status, anaemia) all have an impact on prognosis in RCC.

WHO / ISUP Grading Classification

ISUP developed a grading system for renal tumours in 2012, which was later adopted by the WHO in 2016, validated for prognostication of RCC. [34]

Based on nucleolar prominence and eosinophilia

Table 20 – WHO / ISUP grading classification for renal tumours [35]

Grade	Description
1	Nucleoli absent or inconspicuous at x400 magnification
2	Nucleoli conspicuous and eosinophilic at x400 magnification and visible but not prominent at x100 magnification
3	Nucleoli are conspicuous and eosinophilic at x100 magnification
4	Extreme nuclear pleomorphism, multi-nucleate giant cells and / or rhabdoid and / or sarcomatoid differentiation

Leibovich Scoring System

The Leibovich scoring system is used to predict a patient with RCC risk of developing metastatic disease after RN. [36]

The risk categories are stratified as follows:

- Low risk: 0–2 points
- Intermediate risk: 3–5 points
- High risk: ≥ 6 points

Metastasis-free survival at 10 years is 90% (low risk), 60% (intermediate risk) and 25% (high risk).

Table 21 – Leibovich scoring system for risk stratification of RCC after RN

	Score
T – stage	
pT1a	0
pT1b	2
pT2	3
pT3–4	4
Tumour size (cm)	
< 10cm	0
> 10cm	1
Regional lymph node(s)	
No nodes	0
Node(s) positive	2
Nuclear Grade	
Grade 1–2	0
Grade 3	1
Grade 4	3
Tumour necrosis	
None	0
Present	1

TREATMENT

NEPHRON-SPARING SURGERY

There are various indications for undergoing partial nephrectomy (PN):
- *absolute*, single (functioning) kidney, bilateral synchronous RCC
- *relative*, unilateral RCC with poorly functioning contra-lateral kidney and/or co-morbid conditions predisposing to kidney disease (e.g. diabetes), increased risk of secondary malignancy (e.g. hereditary, VHL)
- *elective*, localised unilateral RCC with normal contra-lateral kidney (T1 < 7cm)

Small tumours near the hilum, poor renal parenchyma and renal vein thrombosis may make a patient unsuitable for PN.

The patient must be consented for the need for open conversion (0.5–2%), conversion to radical nephrectomy (2–10%), bleeding requiring embolization (2–10%), urine leak (0.5–2%).

Most common complication after PN for endophytic tumours is urine leak – this can be managed with antibiotics, stent insertion and leaving drain in situ.

EAU recommends PN should be offered to all suitable patients with T1 tumours. [31]

PN has been shown to better preserve kidney function.

The risks of bleeding are greater than radical nephrectomy (RN).

Positive surgical margin present in 8% of PN patients (higher than for RN), however remains unclear whether has adverse impact on CSS and re-resection is not routinely indicated.

Oncological outcomes of open vs. laparoscopic vs. Robot-assisted PN are comparable.

Open technique has shorter operative time, longer in-patient stay, greater blood loss.

Steps for PN

The broad steps for performing PN for the FRCS (Urol) viva are as follows:
- GA, prepped and draped in lateral position and upward arc
- all facets of WHO checklist complete
- mobilise bowel, free up upper and lower poles and de-fat the kidney
- identify the tumours and delineate these
- clamp vessels and start timer
- excise tumour > 1mm margin, close any collecting system injury with absorbable sutures and surgicel, drain placement (+/- stent)

RENAL / PADUA Scores

PN is a challenging operation and scoring systems have been devised to predict the peri-operative complications of this procedure. [37]

Both RENAL and / or PADUA scores can be used, as they both broadly focus on radiological anatomical features and tumour size.

The PADUA score is detailed in (Table 22) and (Image 2).

The renal sinus was defined as the cavity surrounded by kidney parenchyma, lined by capsule and almost filled by renal vessels and pelvis with the remaining space filled by fat. [38]

Original PADUA study reported 30x complication risk if PADUA score ≥ 10p compared to 6–7p. [38]

Table 22 – PADUA scoring system for predicting perioperative complications during PN

	1 point	2 points	3 points
Maximum radius (cm)	≤ 4	4–7	≥ 7
Exo- / Endo- phytic	≥ 50% exophytic	< 50% exophytic	Entirely endophytic
Location to sinus line	Entirely above / below or < 50% crossing	> 50% crossing or entirely between lines	
Renal rim	Lateral	Medial	
Renal sinus	No relationship	Renal sinus location	
Collecting system	Not involved	Infiltrated	

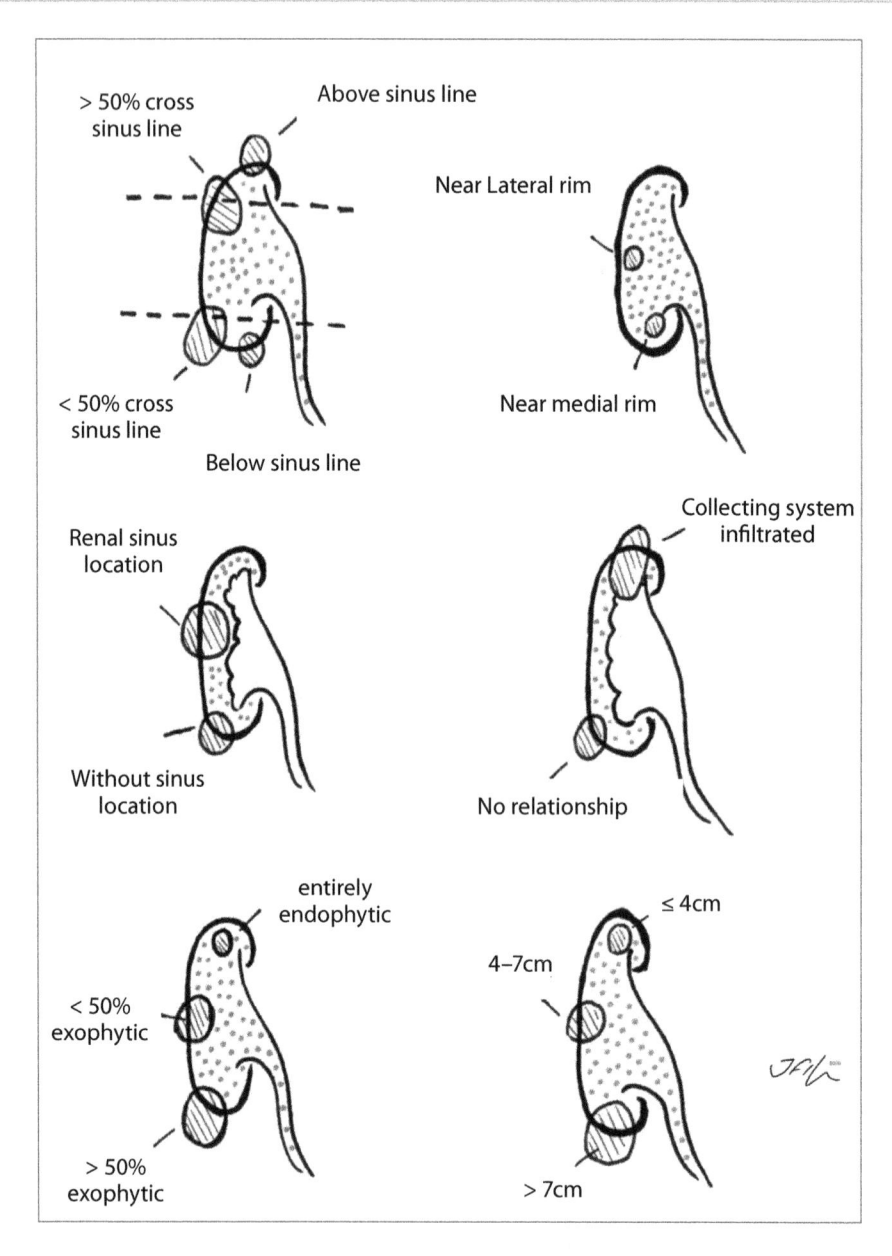

Image 2 – PADUA scoring system for perioperative complications in PN

RADICAL NEPHRECTOMY

Remains gold-standard operation to treat T2–4 RCC and T1 unsuitable for PN.

Involves excising the kidney with all the tumour, Gerota's fascia +/- adrenalectomy +/- LND.

Laparoscopic vs. open RN have comparable oncological outcomes, however laparoscopic has shorter in-patient stay, lower blood loss and morbidity and greater operative time.

Retro- or intra-peritoneal approaches have similar oncological outcomes and QOL variables.

Retro- vs. Trans- Peritoneal RN

There is no difference in oncological outcomes between retro- and trans-peritoneal RN. [31]

Retroperitoneal approach allows early visualisation of the renal artery, reduced risk of injury to organs in peritoneal cavity and any bleeding is contained within retroperitoneal cavity.

Transperitoneal allows more space for operative working field.

Adrenalectomy

Ipsilateral adrenalectomy in the absence of radiological / intra-operatively evident adrenal gland involvement, has no survival advantage and is not indicated.

Only perform if pre-operative imaging suggests adrenal involvement (or found intra-operatively).

Lymph Node Dissection

The indication for LND together with PN or RN remains controversial.

If clinically enlarged then a LND may be considered for staging purposes.

CT / MRI cannot distinguish a metastatic from normal node if the size is normal, and < 20% of dissected suspicious nodes during RN are positive for metastatic disease on histology.

Currently in patients with localised disease without evidence of LN metastasis, performing LND in conjunction with RN confers no benefit to CSS or OS.

Renal Artery Embolization

Embolization of the renal artery can be undertaken hours before RN.

This procedure can reduce blood loss, allow ligation of the renal vein first and facilitate dissection due to tissue oedema.

"Post-infarction syndrome" is the most common complication – pain, nausea, fever.

ACTIVE SURVEILLANCE

AS defined as the initial monitoring of tumour size by serial abdominal imaging (US, CT, MRI) with delayed intervention reserved for tumours showing clinical progression.

Watchful waiting implies that patient co-morbidities preclude any future treatment and therefore tumours do not require follow-up imaging.

Largest series of AS found growth of renal tumours was low and metastatic progression 1–2%. [39]

Overall, both short- and intermediate- term oncological outcomes indicate that in selected frail / co-morbid patients, AS is initially appropriate to monitor small renal masses.

Lower long-term cancer-specific mortality for patients undergoing surgery.

CRYOSURGERY (CS)

For tumours < 4 cm in size

Usually performed under GA, the kidney can be accessed CT-guided (percutaneous), loin incision (open) or laparoscopically +/- concurrent renal biopsy.

Involves direct insertion of freezing probes into tumour and two separate freeze / thaw cycles resulting in the formation of an "ice-ball".

Complication rates are comparable for percutaneous vs. laparoscopic techniques.

Complications of cryotherapy include:
- infection, pain and bleeding requiring transfusion
- need for further treatment
- pneumothorax requiring insertion of chest drain
- injury to liver, spleen, pancreas, bowel, major vessels

Cryotherapy vs. RFA appear comparable for oncological outcomes (OS, CSS, RFS) and complication rates.

Cryotherapy vs. PN have mixed results in terms of oncological outcomes and complication rates.

AS, RFA or cryotherapy should all be offered to elderly +/- co-morbid patients with small renal masses.

RADIO-FREQUENCY ABLATION

For tumours < 4 cm in size.

Usually performed percutaneously under local anaesthetic (+/- sedation) however occasionally under GA if laparoscopic.

Similar technical principles to cryotherapy, however CT-guided imaging to place the electrode probes which create radio-frequency energy to heat the tumour and kill cancer cells.

Complications are similar to those listed for cryotherapy.

Following RFA the most reliable method of determining success is via CT / MRI with contrast which should demonstrate a shrinkage in size and reduction of tumour enhancement.

FOLLOW-UP

There is no strong evidence to support any particular surveillance scheme, nor for how long follow-up imaging should last for.

Late metastases are likely to be solitary and more amenable to aggressive treatment, reinforcing the notion of prolonged follow-up.

No surveillance regimens have been validated or defined for ablative therapies.

Risk stratification after PN / RN is necessary to predict prognosis and plan a follow-up schedule, and there are many different stratification programmes.

For clear cell RCC, the Leibovich scoring system is used.

The follow up schedule is the same for PN and RN.

EAU 2019 proposed a lifelong surveillance schedule for RCC. [40]

Table 23 – EAU 2019 surveillance schedule following treatment for RCC

Risk Profile					
	6 months	1 year	2 years	3 years	> 3 years
Low risk	US	CT	US	CT	CT every 2 years
Intermediate / High risk	CT	CT	CT	CT	CT every 2 years

METASTATIC RCC

25% of patients newly diagnosed with RCC will harbour metastases at presentation, a further 30% progress to metastases after nephrectomy.

The International Metastatic RCC Database Consortium may be used as prognostic risk stratification in mRCC and determining available treatment options.

Table 24 – International Metastatic RCC Database Consortium prognostic factors and risk categories for mRCC [41]

Prognostic Factor	Cut-off Point
Karnofsky performance status	< 80
Time from diagnosis to treatment	< 12 months
Haemoglobin	< LLN
Neutrophil	> ULN
Corrected serum calcium	> ULN
Platelet	> ULN

Risk Category	Factors Present
Good prognosis	0–1
Intermediate prognosis	2
Poor prognosis	> 2

Cytoreductive Nephrectomy

For most patients with mRCC, CN is palliative and systemic treatments are necessary.

For select patients with oligo-metastases, CN can be curative if all deposits are excised.

Embolization

Renal artery embolization is an option for patients with persisting haematuria unfit for surgery.

Embolization to hyper-vascular bone or spinal metastases can reduce intra-operative blood loss during their resection.

Chemotherapy

Do not offer chemotherapy as first-line therapy in patients with metastatic clear-cell RCC.

There is weak evidence of benefit of gemcitabine + doxorubicin in sarcomatoid RCC.

Immunotherapy

IFN-alpha has conflicting evidence of benefit in mRCC, it should not be used as monotherapy.

Has been superseded by targeted therapies in mRCC.

Tyrosine-Kinase Inhibitors (TKIs)

Part of the group of targeted therapies in mRCC – have suffix -ib. (e.g. sunitinib, axitinib).

Tyrosine kinases are enzymes responsible for the activation of proteins by signal transduction cascades (phosphorylation – adding a phosphate group to the protein) which TKIs inhibit.

Anti-angiogenic agents that target the VEGF pathway include sunitinib and pazopanib – and are first line targeted treatment in mRCC.

Renal cancer sub-type most likely to benefit from TKI are clear cell RCC.

For patients who progress on first-line VEGF therapy (VEGF resistant disease).

CARMENA study evaluated 450 mRCC patients to TKI drug sunitinib alone vs. CN + sunitinib (1:1) with the primary end point of the study being OS. [42]

sunitinib non-inferior when used alone for intermediate and poor risk mRCC disease

mTOR Inhibitors

Drugs that inhibit the rapamycin target (a protein kinase) – have the suffix -imus (e.g. temsirolimus).

BENIGN RENAL MASSES

POLYCYSTIC KIDNEY DISEASE

Autosomal dominant, associated with development of multiple expanding bilateral parenchymal cysts, commonly presents 30–40 years and leads to 10% of all cases of ESRF.

- associated with Berry aneurysms, hepatic cysts, diverticulosis and mitral valve prolapse
- genetic defect located on short arm of chromosome 16 and PKD2 gene on chromosome 4

Autosomal recessive, is much rarer and distinct from ADPKD as it presents in-utero or childhood, with bilateral renal parenchyma enlargement replaced by radially orientated cysts.

- associated with biliary dysgenesis, pulmonary hypoplasia, oligohydramnios

ACQUIRED RENAL CYSTIC DISEASE

Condition occurring in patients with ESRF – particularly on dialysis treatment – as a result of prolonged high levels of nitrogen-containing compounds in the blood (azotaemia).

It is a feature of ESRF rather than being caused by its treatment.

Cysts that burst can result in pain and visible haematuria requiring embolisation.

The association of RCC and dialysis treatment is due to the malignant transformation of ARCD cysts, with the cut-off of 3 cm in size raising suspicion for RCC.

MULTI-CYSTIC DYSPLASTIC KIDNEY

Can be sporadic or inherited in autosomal dominant manner.

More common unilaterally, bilateral disease is lethal. Associated with contra-lateral PUJ obstruction (10%) and reflux.

Irregular collection of tense non-communicating cysts lined with cuboidal tubular epithelium and dysplastic renal parenchyma.

4x increased risk of malignancy (Wilm's tumour, not RCC) however prophylactic nephrectomy is not recommended unless for treating refractory hypertension (rare).

Almost always associated with ureteric atresia / obstruction.

MULTI-LOCULAR CYST (CYSTIC NEPHROMA)

More common in females and demonstrate bi-modal age distribution.

Benign cysts tend to be bulky with thick capsules and highly echogenic septa – aspiration yield yellow fluid with solid elements.

Range from benign to Wilm's tumour to cystic RCC – surgical excision recommended.

ONCOCYTOMA

Oncocytoma is the most common benign solid renal tumour (5% of all renal tumours) and tends to affect the elderly.

Most are diagnosed incidentally, however can present with flank pain, haematuria, palpable mass.

They cannot be distinguished radiologically from RCC, signs for oncocytoma:

- central stellate scar (CT / MRI)
- spoke-wheel pattern of feeding arteries (angiography)

Macroscopically they are spherical, homogenous tan-coloured lesions.

Microscopically they do not have any malignant features (e.g. invasion, metastases, lymphadenopathy) and are uniform eosinophilic cells packed with mitochondria.

Biopsy is not recommended because oncocytoma and RCC can co-exist, as well as eosinophilic variant of chromophobe RCC can be difficult to distinguish from oncocytoma on biopsy.

Treatment is surgical excision by PN or RN, however after histological confirmation patients do not need to be followed up.

UPPER TRACT UROTHELIAL CANCER

EPIDEMIOLOGY

Upper tract urothelial carcinomas (UTUC) (TCC) are uncommon constituting 5% of all urothelial cancers.

Pelvi-calyceal TCC twice as common as ureteric TCC (half of these are multi-focal and most are distal).

Kidney TCCs constitute 10% of the total number of kidney cancers. [1]

17% of patients with UTUC will also present with tumour in the bladder, whilst recurrence in the bladder after UTUC treatment is 25%.

There is familial UTUC linked to hereditary non-polyposis colorectal carcinoma (HNPCC) and this should be screened for at initial presentation.

RISK FACTORS

Age	peak incidence age 70–90 years
Gender	3x more common in men
Tobacco	2–7x increased relative risk [43]
Occupation	aromatic amine exposure (rubber and dye manufacturing, pesticides)
HNPCC	(Lynch syndrome) is a cancer syndrome associated with UTUC
Drugs	phenacetin (NSAID no longer in use), aristolochic acid (Chinese herbal medicine)
Genetic	chromosome 9, 17 (p53 loci) and 13 (retinoblastoma gene)

DIAGNOSIS

SYMPTOMS

The most common symptom is painless visible haematuria.

IMAGING

CTU has the highest diagnostic accuracy for UTUC of all imaging techniques.

- secondary sign of hydronephrosis is a poor prognostic sign
- enlarged local LN is highly predictive of metastasis

CTU is preferable to MRU.

MRU (gadolinium-based contrast) is an alternative to CTU for patients contra-indicated to radiation or iodinated contrast media, however not suitable if eGFR < 30 mL /min.

CYTOLOGY

Should preferably be performed "selectively" in situ, with a ureteric catheter collecting during ureteroscopy (prior to retrograde study which can cause deterioration of sample).

DIAGNOSTIC URETEROSCOPY

This should be used in scenarios of clinical uncertainty or when kidney-sparing surgery is considered such as single kidney.

BAUS review found 80% of nephro-ureterectomies did not have prior histological diagnosis (and almost all specimens confirmed malignancy). [1]

Under-staging with ureteroscopic biopsies is common.

STAGING

The majority of UTUCs are invasive at diagnosis (60%) when compared to bladder tumours (15%).

Concurrent bladder tumours with UTUC are common (17%) and recurrences in the bladder after UTUC treatment occur in 22–47%.

Synchronous and metachronous UTUCs occur in 3% approximately, highlighting the importance of surveillance (cystoscopic, radiological and cytological) for these patients.

Table 25 – TNM staging classification for UTUC [43]

T – Primary Tumour	
TX	Primary tumour cannot be assessed
T0	No evidence of primary tumour
Ta	Non-invasive papillary carcinoma
Tis	Carcinoma in situ
T1	Tumour invades sub-epithelial connective tissue
T2	Tumour invades muscularis
T3	(renal pelvis) – tumour invades beyond muscularis into peripelvic fat or renal parenchyma
	(ureter) – tumour invades beyond muscularis into periureteric fat
T4	Tumour invades adjacent organs or through the kidney into perinephric
N – Lymph nodes	
NX	Regional lymph nodes cannot be assessed
N0	No regional lymph node metastasis
N1	Metastasis in single lymph node ≤ 2cm in greatest dimension
N2	Metastasis in single lymph node > 2cm in greatest dimension or multiple lymph nodes
M – Metastasis	
M0	No distant metastasis
M1	Distant metastasis

TREATMENT

KIDNEY SPARING SURGERY

KSS for low-risk UTUC spares the patient from the morbidity of major surgery, without compromising renal function or oncological outcome.

In low-risk disease (uni-focal tumour, < 1cm size, low-grade, no invasion on CTU) survival is similar between KSS and radical nephroureterectomy (RNU). [43]

KSS should be considered as primary approach in all low-risk tumours, and in imperative cases for high-risk disease (e.g. single kidney, chronic renal impairment). [43]

Partial nephrectomy is not considered an option in treating UTUC.

Ureteroscopic Ablation

LASER fulguration of tumour base by Holmium : YAG or Nd : YAG LASERs

Retrograde stenting is required.

Percutaneous Access

Disrupts urothelial integrity and is more invasive however it allows excellent access to renal pelvis with 30 Fr sheath to ablate / resect tumour.

Allows delivery of adjuvant therapy such as MMC or BCG.

Isolated Distal Ureteric Tumour

Gold-standard treatment is RNU with excision of cuff of bladder tissue, however a ureteric segmental resection has a role where renal preservation is paramount (e.g. single kidney).

Option is spatulated tension-free uretero-ureteral anastomosis.

RADICAL NEPHROURETERECTOMY

Cystoscopy prior to RNU must be undertaken to rule out bladder tumour.

RNU with bladder cuff excision is the standard treatment for UTUC regardless of its location.

Open RNU can be done entirely through a midline incision, or with a loin incision and a second Pfannensteil or lower midline incision for the cuff.

Laparoscopic vs. Open RNU have been shown to be comparable in outcome and safety.

(T3 and high-grade disease should be treated by open surgery.)

The distal ureter can be mobilised via the "rip and pluck" technique, whereby the distal ureter is cystoscopically resected down to peri-vesical fat and then plucked during dissection. Benefit is avoiding second incision; drawback is potential tumour cell spillage.

LND should not be performed for TaT1 disease.

Due to the high risk of bladder recurrence after UTUC treatment (22–47%), EAU recommends that SI MMC intra-vesical be given post-operatively. [43]

CHEMO-RADIO THERAPY

Radiotherapy has no role in the management of UTUC.

POUT trial was a RCT evaluating role of chemotherapy in UTUC.

Patients with UTUC, WHO performance status 0–1 and undergoing RNU were randomised 1 : 1 to post-operative surveillance vs. adjuvant cisplatin-based chemotherapy (4 cycles).

Primary end-point was disease free survival at 3 years (71% treatment arm vs. 46% surveillance). [44]

FOLLOW-UP

Close follow-up of UTUC is essential to monitor for metachronous bladder and contra-lateral ureteric recurrences (cystoscopy, cytology, CTU).

Flexible cystoscopy and cytology – at 3 months and then annually

CTU – annually for non-invasive tumours, 6-monthly for 2 years for invasive tumours then annually

For patients who have undergone KSS, the follow-up should be more intense and therefore relies on significant patient compliance.

3 months – cytology, CTU and ureteroscopy

6 months – cytology, CTU and ureteroscopy (URS repeated at 12, 18, 24, 30 months)

Then annually all 3 should be undertaken.

METASTATIC DISEASE

Carries a poor prognosis.

After discussion at MDT, palliative care input should be offered.

There is no current evidence supporting the benefit of chemotherapy for such patients.

There is no current evidence supporting the role of metastasectomy.

REFERENCES

1. Mak D, Khan MJ, Fernando HS. Urothelial cancer. In: Arya M, Shergill IS, Fernando HS et al. (2018) Viva Practice for the FRCS(Urol) and Postgraduate Urology Examinations 2nd Edition, CRC Press, London.
2. Pareek G, Shevchuk M, Armenakas NA, et al. (2003). The effect of finasteride on the expression of vascular endothelial growth factor and microvessel density: a possible mechanism for decreased prostatic bleeding in treated patients. *The Journal of urology*, *169*(1), 20–23.
3. Britton JP, Dowell AC, Whelan P, (1992). A community study of bladder cancer screening by the detection of occult urinary bleeding. *The Journal of urology*, *148*(3 Part 1), 788–790.
4. Messing EM, Madeb RR, Golijanin D. (2006). 881: Long-Term Outcome of Hematuria Home Screening for Bladder Cancer (BC). *The Journal of Urology*, *175*(4S), 284–285.
5. Khadra MH, Pickard RS, Charlton M, (2000). A prospective analysis of 1,930 patients with hematuria to evaluate current diagnostic practice. *The Journal of urology*, *163*(2), 524–527.
6. NICE guideline: Suspected cancer: recognition and referral. Available at: https://www.nice.org.uk/guidance/ng12/resources/suspected-cancer-recognition-and-referral-pdf-1837268071621 [last accessed 28 May 2020].
7. Price SJ, Shephard EA, Stapley SA, et al. (2014). Non-visible versus visible haematuria and bladder cancer risk: a study of electronic records in primary care. *British Journal of General Practice*, *64*(626), e584–e589.
8. Joint Consensus Statement on the Initial Assessment of Haematuria (2008). Available at: https://www.baus.org.uk/_userfiles/pages/files/News/haematuria_consensus_guidelines_July_2008.pdf [last accessed on 27 May 2020].
9. Babjuk M, Burger M, Comperat E, (2018) EAU Guidelines on Non-muscle-invasive Bladder Cancer (TaT1 and CIS). Available at: https://uroweb.org/wp-content/uploads/EAU-Guidelines-Non-muscle-invasive-Bladder-Cancer-TaT1-CIS-2018.pdf [last accessed 28 May 2020].
10. Montironi R, Lopez-Beltran A. (2005). The 2004 WHO classification of bladder tumors: a summary and commentary. *International journal of surgical pathology*, *13*(2), 143–153.
11. NICE: Managing non-muscle-invasive bladder cancer (2020). Available at: https://pathways.nice.org.uk/pathways/bladder-cancer/managing-muscle-invasive-bladder-cancer [last accessed 29 May 2020].

12. Sylvester RJ, Oosterlinck W, Holmang S, et al. (2016). Systematic review and individual patient data meta-analysis of randomized trials comparing a single immediate instillation of chemotherapy after transurethral resection with transurethral resection alone in patients with stage pTa–pT1 urothelial carcinoma of the bladder: which patients benefit from the instillation?. *European urology*, *69*(2), 231–244.
13. Sylvester RJ, van der Meijden AP, Lamm DL. (2002). Intravesical bacillus Calmette-Guerin reduces the risk of progression in patients with superficial bladder cancer: a meta-analysis of the published results of randomized clinical trials. *The Journal of urology*, *168*(5), 1964–1970.
14. Boorjian SA, Kim SP, Tollefson MK, (2013). Comparative performance of comorbidity indices for estimating perioperative and 5-year all-cause mortality following radical cystectomy for bladder cancer. *The Journal of urology*, *190*(1), 55–60.
15. Johnston MC, Marks A, Crilly MA, (2015) Charlson index scores from administrative data and case-note review compared favourably in a renal disease cohort. *The European Journal of Public Health*, *25*(3), 391–396.
16. Witjes JA, Bruins M, Cathomas R, et al. (2019) EAU Guidelines on Muscle-invasive and Metastatic Bladder Cancer. Available at: https://uroweb.org/wp-content/uploads/EAU-Guidelines-on-Muscle-invasive-and-Metastatic-Bladder-Cancer-2019.pdf [last accessed on 30 May 2020].
17. NICE: Appendix C, WHO performance status classification. Available at: https://www.nice.org.uk/guidance/ta121/chapter/Appendix-C-WHO-performance-status-classification [last accessed 30 May 2020].
18. Agnew N. (2010). Preoperative cardiopulmonary exercise testing. *Continuing education in anaesthesia, critical care & pain*, *10*(2), 33–37.
19. Vale CL. (2005). Neoadjuvant chemotherapy in invasive bladder cancer: update of a systematic review and meta-analysis of individual patient data: Advanced Bladder Cancer (ABC) Meta-analysis Collaboration. *European urology*, *48*(2), 202–206.
20. NICE: Managing muscle-invasive bladder cancer (2020). Available at: https://pathways.nice.org.uk/pathways/bladder-cancer/managing-muscle-invasive-bladder-cancer [last accessed 30 May 2020].
21. Lonser RR, Glenn GM, Walther M, (2003). von Hippel-Lindau disease. *The Lancet*, *361*(9374), 2059–2067.
22. Menko FH, Van Steensel MA, Giraud S, et al. (2009). Birt-Hogg-Dubé syndrome: diagnosis and management. *The Lancet Oncology*, *10*(12), 1199–1206.

23. Haas NB, Nathanson KL, (2014). Hereditary kidney cancer syndromes. *Advances in chronic kidney disease*, *21*(1), 81–90.
24. Koo KC, Kim WT, Ham WS, et al. (2010) Trends of presentation and clinical outcome of treated renal angiomyolipoma. *Yonsei medical journal* 51, no. 5 (2010): 728–734.
25. Luca D, Rossetti R. (1999). Management of renal angiomyolipoma: a report of 53 cases. *BJU international*, *83*(3), 215–218.
26. Crino PB, Nathanson KL, Henske EP, (2006). The tuberous sclerosis complex. *New England Journal of Medicine*, *355*(13), 1345–1356.
27. Medda M, Picozzi SC, Bozzini G, (2009). Wunderlich's syndrome and hemorrhagic shock. *Journal of Emergencies, Trauma and Shock*, *2*(3), 203.
28. Maheshwari E, O'Malley ME, Ghai S, (2010). Split-bolus MDCT urography: upper tract opacification and performance for upper tract tumors in patients with hematuria. *American Journal of Roentgenology*, *194*(2), 453–458.
29. Bromwich E, Qteishat A, Fernando HS et al. (2018) In: Viva Practice for the FRCS(Urol) and Postgraduate Urology Examinations 2nd Edition, CRC Press, London.
30. Marconi L, Dabestani S, Lam TB, (2016). Systematic review and meta-analysis of diagnostic accuracy of percutaneous renal tumour biopsy. *European urology*, *69*(4), 660–673.
31. Ljungberg B, Albiges L, Bensalah K, et al. (2018) EAU Guidelines on Renal Cell Carcinoma. Available at: https://uroweb.org/wp-content/uploads/EAU-RCC-Guidelines-2018-large-text.pdf [last accessed 30 May 2020].
32. Adams LC, Ralla B, Bender YNY, et al. (2018) Renal cell carcinoma with venous extension: prediction of inferior vena cava wall invasion by MRI. *Cancer Imaging*, *18*(1), 17.
33. Sweeney P, Wood CG, Pisters LL, et al. (2003) Surgical management of renal cell carcinoma associated with complex inferior vena caval thrombi. Urol Oncol; 21: 327–33.
34. Delahunt B, Eble JN, Egevad L, (2019). Grading of renal cell carcinoma. *Histopathology*, *74*(1), 4–17.
35. Moch H. (2016) The WHO/ISUP grading system for renal carcinoma. *Der Pathologe*, *37*(4), 355–360.
36. Leibovich BC, Blute ML, Cheville JC, et al. (2003) Prediction of progression after radical nephrectomy for patients with clear cell renal cell carcinoma: a stratification tool for prospective clinical trials. *Cancer: Interdisciplinary International Journal of the American Cancer Society*, *97*(7), 1663–1671.

37. Hew MN, Baseskioglu B, Barwari K, et al. (2011). Critical appraisal of the PADUA classification and assessment of the RENAL nephrometry score in patients undergoing partial nephrectomy. *The Journal of urology*, 186(1), 42–46.
38. Ficarra V, Novara G, Secco S, et al. (2009) Preoperative aspects and dimensions used for an anatomical (PADUA) classification of renal tumours in patients who are candidates for nephron-sparing surgery. *European urology*, 56(5), 786–793.
39. Jewett MA, Mattar K, Basiuk J, et al. (2011). Active surveillance of small renal masses: progression patterns of early stage kidney cancer. *European urology*, 60(1), 39–44.
40. Ljungberg B, Albiges L, Bensalah K, et al. (2019) EAU Guidelines on Renal Cell Carcinoma. Available at: https://uroweb.org/wp-content/uploads/EAU-Pocket-Guidelines-Renal-Cell-Carcinoma-2019.pdf [last accessed 29 May 2020].
41. Ko JJ, Xie W, Kroeger N, et al. (2015). The International Metastatic Renal Cell Carcinoma Database Consortium model as a prognostic tool in patients with metastatic renal cell carcinoma previously treated with first-line targeted therapy: a population-based study. *The Lancet oncology*, 16(3), 293–300.
42. Méjean A, Ravaud A, Thezenas S, et al. (2018). Sunitinib alone or after nephrectomy in metastatic renal-cell carcinoma. *New England Journal of Medicine*, 379(5), 417–427.
43. Roupret M, Babjuk M, Burger M et al. (2019) EAU Guidelines on Upper Urinary Tract Urothelial Carcinoma. Available at: https://uroweb.org/wp-content/uploads/EAU-Guidelines-on-Upper-urinary-Tract-Tumours-2019.pdf [last accessed 30 May 2020].
44. Birtle A, Johnson M, Chester J, et al. (2020). Adjuvant chemotherapy in upper tract urothelial carcinoma (the POUT trial): a phase 3, open-label, randomised controlled trial. *The Lancet* 395(10232), 1268–1277.

UROLOGICAL ONCOLOGY 1 MCQS

1. Which of the following tests has not been explored as a potential marker for detecting urothelial cancer in urine?
   A) uroVysion
   B) BSP
   C) BTA stat
   D) ImmunoCyt
   E) UBC test

2. Which of the following statements regarding PDD cystoscopy is false?
   A) under blue light, healthy bladder may appear red
   B) 5-ALA is converted to haem in cytoplasm of urothelial cells
   C) the trigone often fluoresces without malignant pathology
   D) blue light has wavelength of 375–440nm
   E) resection of a blue light abnormal area should be undertaken under white light

3. Which of the following measurements is not routinely taken during CPEX testing?
   A) tidal volume (TV)
   B) residual volume (RV)
   C) 12 lead ECG
   D) respiratory exchange ratio (RER)
   E) non-invasive arterial pressure (NIAP)

4. On which chromosome is the VHL gene found?
   A) 3
   B) 5
   C) 7
   D) 9
   E) 11

5. A newly diagnosed patient with RCC has a 7.5cm right sided kidney tumour, with staging CT TAP revealing extension into the surrounding perirenal fat and contiguous adrenal gland, hilar lymph nodes are normal.

   What is the correct TNM staging for this patient?

   A) T3aN0M1
   B) T3bN0M0
   C) T3cN0M1
   D) T4N0M0
   E) T4N0M1

6. Which of the following statements regarding the CARMENA trial is true?

   A) axitinib group was compared to axitinib + CN group in 1 : 1 randomisation
   B) the primary end point of the study was disease free survival
   C) patients on anti-coagulants were excluded
   D) the dose of axitinib was 50mg once daily
   E) axinitib alone was non inferior to axitinib + CN in the primary end point of the study

7. The histology from a radical nephrectomy report reads as: eosinophilic cells packed with mitochondria, acidophilic cytoplasm, microscopic nested architecture, myxoid stroma and areas of degenerative cytologic atypia.

   Which is the most likely underlying renal tumour that has been excised?

   A) leiomyosarcoma
   B) chromophobe RCC
   C) oncocytoma
   D) papillary type 1 tumour
   E) papillary type 2 tumour

8. A newly diagnosed patient with UTUC has undergone RNU and full staging CT. The primary tumour invades the renal parenchyma, a single positive lymph node of 3cm has been excised and there is no distant metastasis.

   What is the correct TNM staging for this patient?

   A) T3aN1M0
   B) T3aN2M0
   C) T3N1M0
   D) T3N2M0
   E) T4N1M0

9. Which of the following is not a parameter as part of the International Metastatic RCC Database Consortium risk stratification tool?
   A) neutrophil count
   B) serum calcium
   C) haemoglobin
   D) platelet count
   E) time from diagnosis to treatment < 6 months

10. A newly diagnosed patient with 9cm renal tumour has thrombus extending into the IVC 3cm above the level of the renal vein orifice.
    Which of the following statements is true?
    A) this is T3b disease
    B) this is level 3 IVC involvement
    C) this is level 4 IVC involvement
    D) cardiopulmonary bypass may be required for operative intervention
    E) histology will most likely have be papillary carcinoma

11. Which of the following is not a parameter on the Leibovich scoring system for risk stratification in RCC?
    A) tumour necrosis
    B) tumour size
    C) tumour grade
    D) T-stage
    E) sarcomatoid differentiation

12. Which of the following is not a recognised paraneoplastic symptom or syndrome associated with RCC?
    A) polycythaemia
    B) Waldenstrom's macroglobulinemia
    C) Cushing's syndrome
    D) galactorrhea
    E) amyloidosis

13. On which chromosome does the gene mutation responsible for BHD occur?
    A) 13
    B) 15
    C) 17
    D) 19
    E) 21

14. Which of the following statements regarding ileal conduit urinary diversion in radical cystectomy is false?
    A) 15cm of ileum should be used
    B) post-operative metabolic acidosis is less common than in neobladder formation
    C) Bricker technique involves spatulating and anastomosing each ureter to the serosa of the bowel separately
    D) Wallace 1 technique involves suturing the lateral walls of the spatulated ureters and anastomosing these to the anti-mesenteric part of the open bowel segment
    E) Entero-ureteric stricture rates between Wallace 1 and Bricker techniques are comparable

15. Which of the following statements regarding lymph node dissection in radical cystectomy is false?
    A) extended LND involves taking lymph nodes up to the inferior mesenteric artery
    B) 5-year CSS with positive nodal involvement is 40%
    C) 3 positive nodes in presacral group equates to N-stage 2 in TNM staging classification
    D) post-operative pain and paraesthesia down the medial thigh suggest obturator nerve injury
    E) anti-coagulation with LMWH can cause prolonged lymphorrhea

16. Conventional total dose of fractionated radiation in EBRT for MIBC is:
    A) 25–35 Gy
    B) 35–45 Gy
    C) 45–60 Gy
    D) 60–70 Gy
    E) 70–80 Gy

17. Which of the following statements regarding the POUT trial is true?
    A) there is an agreed international consensus on benefit of adjuvant chemotherapy for UTUC
    B) node positive patients were excluded from the trial
    C) patients with oligo metastasis were included in the trial
    D) chemotherapy had to be given within < 90 days of RNU
    E) patients with performance status ≤ 2 were included in the trial

18. Which of the following statements regarding AML is false?
    A) AML are the most common benign mesenchymal tumour
    B) 30% are due to tuberous sclerosis
    C) familial AML grow faster than sporadic AML
    D) everolimus is used to reduce AML volume in tuberous sclerosis
    E) vascular component is in the form of thick-walled hyalinized vessels

19. A full course of BCG (e.g. Lamm's regime) consists of how many doses of intra-vesical BCG?
    A) 17
    B) 19
    C) 21
    D) 24
    E) 27

20. What is the ARR of recurrence of bladder cancer by giving single instillation dose of MMC after first TURBT?
    A) 6%
    B) 8%
    C) 12%
    D) 14%
    E) 16%

21. Which of the following is not a factor used to predict bladder cancer progression and recurrence in NMIBC, in the EORTC scoring system?
    A) tumour necrosis
    B) presence of CIS
    C) prior recurrence rate
    D) tumour grade
    E) tumour multi-focality

22. Which of the following regarding urachal tumours is false?
    A) the majority of cases are adenocarcinomas
    B) it is more common in men
    C) 5-year survival with RC ≤ 70%
    D) tumours with polypoid configuration are more likely to seed
    E) the urachus is a fibrous remnant of the allantois and lies in the space of Retzius

23. Which statement is correct regarding nephrological causes of visible haematuria?
    A) Goodpasture's disease is an auto-immune condition where antibodies attack Bowman's capsule in the kidney
    B) Alport's syndrome involves a Y-linked collagen mutation
    C) Henoch-Schonlein purpura is a systemic vasculitis characterised by deposition of immunoglobulin-A complexes
    D) nephrotic syndrome is associated with raised serum albumin
    E) Berger's disease involves deposition of IgG after a viral upper respiratory tract infection

24. Which statement regarding intra-vesical BCG therapy is false?
    A) is used intra-venously for gastro-intestinal cancer
    B) attaches to urothelium via laminin receptor
    C) upregulates all of IL-2, IL-6 and IL-8
    D) hepatic disorder is a common side effect
    E) it is contraindicated in HIV

25. Which of the following is not a recognised sequalae noted in patients who have previously undergone RC and urinary diversion?
    A) low cobalamin
    B) hyperkalaemia
    C) megaloblastic anaemia
    D) hypomagnesemia
    E) steatorrhea

STATION 2
UROLOGICAL ONCOLOGY 2

PROSTATE CANCER

TESTICULAR CANCER

PENILE CANCER

URETHRAL CANCER

CONTENTS

PROSTATE CANCER	**85**
EPIDEMIOLOGY	85
RISK FACTORS	85
GENETIC PREDISPOSITIONS	86
SCREENING	88
PATHOLOGY	89
HIGH GRADE PROSTATIC INTRA-EPITHELIAL NEOPLASIA	90
ATYPICAL SMALL ACINAR PROLIFERATION	91
OTHER PROSTATE CANCER SUB-TYPES	91
GLEASON GRADING	91
INTERNATIONAL SOCIETY OF UROLOGICAL PATHOLOGY (2014)	92
PROSTATE SPECIFIC ANTIGEN (PSA)	92
PSA VELOCITY	94
PSA DOUBLING-TIME	94
PSA DENSITY	94
FREE TO TOTAL PSA	94
SUPER-SENSITIVE PSA	94
UPM3 TEST	95
STAGING [1]	95
N-STAGING	96
M-STAGING	97
MRI IN PCA	97
PROSTATE BIOPSY	99
TEMPLATE-GUIDED SATURATION BIOPSY	100
RISK STRATIFICATION	100
TREATMENT	101
WATCHFUL WAITING	101
ACTIVE SURVEILLANCE	102
RADICAL PROSTATECTOMY (RP)	103
RADICAL RADIOTHERAPY	106
BRACHYTHERAPY	109
CRYOTHERAPY	110

HIFU	111
HORMONE THERAPY	111
BILATERAL ORCHIDECTOMY	113
LHRH AGONISTS	113
LHRH ANTAGONISTS	114
ANTI-ANDROGENS	114
OESTROGENS	114
CASTRATE-RESISTANT PCA (CRPC) TREATMENT	115
METASTATIC PCA TREATMENT	115
SALVAGE TREATMENT	118
NHS TARGET	118
TESTICULAR CANCER	**120**
EPIDEMIOLOGY	120
PATHOLOGY	121
TUMOUR MARKERS	125
IMAGING	126
STAGING	127
RADICAL ORCHIDECTOMY	129
STAGE 1 GCT TREATMENT	131
STAGE 1 SEMINOMA	131
STAGE 1 NSGCT	133
STAGE II A/B SEMINOMA TREATMENT	135
STAGE II A / B NON-SEMINOMA TREATMENT	135
STAGE 2C / 3 (METASTATIC) TREATMENT	136
SEMINOMAS	136
NON-SEMINOMAS.	136
RESIDUAL TUMOUR RESECTION	137
FOLLOW UP REGIMENS	137
PROGNOSTIC TABLES	138
PENILE CANCER	**140**
EPIDEMIOLOGY	140
RISK FACTORS	140
PATHOLOGY	140
PRE-MALIGNANT LESIONS	141

STAGING	142
TREATMENT	144
SUPERFICIAL NON-INVASIVE DISEASE (CIS)	145
TREATMENT OF INVASIVE DISEASE CONFINED TO GLANS	145
TREATMENT OF INVASIVE DISEASE	146
SUMMARY OF SURGICAL TREATMENTS FOR PRIMARY LESION [83]	147
REGIONAL LYMPH NODE MANAGEMENT	147
FOLLOW UP REGIMEN	150
URETHRAL CANCER	**151**
EPIDEMIOLOGY	151
RISK FACTORS	151
PATHOLOGY	151
INVESTIGATIONS	152
STAGING	152
TREATMENT	153
REFERENCES	**154**
UROLOGICAL ONCOLOGY 2 MCQS	**161**

PROSTATE CANCER

EPIDEMIOLOGY

PCa second most common cancer in men diagnosed worldwide (14% of all cancers), however is the most common cancer in men in the UK.

47,000+ cases diagnosed in UK yearly – more prevalent in developed countries (disease of old age) and greater incidence in countries with highest rates of screening.

Post-mortem studies – evidence of PCa in 30% of 50 year olds, 70% of 80 year olds.

Lifetime risk 1 in 9, (however only 3% of all male deaths will be due to PCa)

Median age at diagnosis – 66 years

71% of PCa deaths occur > 75 years

Late stage diagnosis is more common in aged > 80 years (56% stage 3–4 at time of diagnosis). [1]

RISK FACTORS

Age 75% of all cancers diagnosed in men > 65 years

(however vit.D deficiency is more common in elderly)

Ethnicity Afro-Caribbean > White > Asians (their migration West increases risk) [2]

higher risk Scandinavia and countries adopting a Westernised diet, proposed association with reduced sunlight exposure + Vit.D

Afro-Caribbean men have relative incidence of 1.6 compared to white men

Hereditary (true only in 9%)

defined as 3+ affected relatives, or 2+ with early onset disease (< 55 years)

single defect on Chromosome 1q (HPC1 locus), 8p (MSR-1 locus) and 13q (BRCA2 gene mutations)

RRx2 (x1 1st degree rel.), RRx4 (x2 1st degree rel.), RRx5 if hereditary

Obesity	lower risk of low-grade PCa, higher risk of high-grade PCa (REDUCE study)
	cholesterol / HDLs / LDLs no risk association, statins do not confer protection against PCa (REDUCE study) [3]
	lower circulating androgens (causing lower PSA) and higher free IGF-1 levels
Exercise	confers protection vs. PCa
	proposed mechanism by reducing IGF-1, insulin, testosterone, stimulates antioxidant pathways to reduce harmful reactive oxygen species
Diet	*increase risk*: dairy (high calcium which suppresses Vit.D), excess/zero alcohol (i.e. J-shape), vit.E (SELECT Trial) [4]
	decrease risk: lycopene (carotene) in tomato (cooked tomato-based foods)
Vit.D	U-shaped relationship with PCa
	polymorphisms result in vit.D receptors with lower activity increasing PCa risk
Testosterone	no reported increased risk when given to hypogonadal men [5]
5ARIs	not approved by EMA for this purpose
	proposed lower incidence of PCa but higher risk of high-grade PCa (PCPT) [6]
Prostatitis	chronic prostatitis or inflammation, STIs, CMV, HPV – impaired ability to combat oxidative stress
IGF-1 level	elevated serum levels of IGF-1 yield higher risk of developing PCa

GENETIC PREDISPOSITIONS

Gene fusions are common in PCa and are fundamental for growth and progression.

Most commonly involves fusion of TMPRSS2 to members of ETS family.

Promotes genes under androgenic control (fusion found in up to 50% cases of primary PCa). [7]

TMPRSS2 related gene fusions are highly specific for PCa.

The TMPRSS2 is prostate specific and expressed in both benign & malignant prostatic epithelium.

A variety of other genes are implicated in PCa:
- cell cycle genes: cyclinD2, 14-3-3
- DNA repair genes: GSTpi, GPX3 and GSTM1
- tumour suppressor genes: APC, RASSF1alpha, DKK3, E-cadherin
- hormonal response genes: ERalphaA, ERbeta, RARbeta

PCPT Trial (2003) – Prostate Cancer Prevention Trial [6]

Recruited 18,000 men with no known evidence of PCa and PSA < 3ng / ml.

Randomised to Placebo vs. Finasteride 5mg OD for < 7 years.

TRUS Biopsy was performed if: rising PSA >4, new abnormal DRE or at end of study.

Placebo arm (24% had PCa) vs. Finasteride arm (18% had PCa) – reduce risk by 25%

Higher incidence of high-grade PCa with Finasteride (6.4%) vs. Placebo (5.1%)

REDUCE Trial (2010) – Reduction of Dutasteride of Prostate Cancer Events [3]

International, multi-centre, double-blind, placebo-controlled chemo-prevention study

Inclusion: negative prostate biopsy within 6 months of entry and PSA 2.5–10 (50–60 years) and PSA 3–10 (>60 years), total of 6700+ patients

TRUS biopsy repeated at 2 and 4 years after entry into trial.

Relative risk reduction of PCa by 22% in dutasteride arm (but higher incidence of high-grade PCa)

SELECT (2011) – Selenium and vitamin E Cancer prevention Trial [4]

Multi-centre trial from North America of 35,000 men

Inclusion: PSA < 4, no PCa suggested by DRE, age > 50 years (black men) and > 55 years (all other men)

Randomly assigned to 4 groups: selenium vs. vit.E vs. (Vit.E + selenium) vs. placebo

Main outcome measure: PCa incidence detection

Finding: vit.E significantly increased PCa incidence (however combination treatment had no effect)

SCREENING

PSA screening for PCa is controversial and does not fulfil all the Wilson and Jungner's criteria for a screening programme as listed below: [8]

Table 1 – Wilson and Jungner classic screening criteria

Condition should be an important health problem
There should be an accepted treatment for patients with disease
Facilities for diagnosis and treatment should be available
There should be a recognisable latent or early symptomatic stage
There should be a suitable test for the disease
The test should be acceptable to the population
The natural history of the condition should be adequately understood
There should be an agreed policy on whom to treat as patients
The cost of case-finding should be balanced in relation to medical care cost as a whole
Case-finding should be a continuing process and not a "once and for all" project

PSA lacks specificity (only 40%) and sensitivity.

PCa has long latent period allowing patients to die from other causes.

The incidence of PCa is highest in countries with the highest uptake of PCa screening.

PLCO Trial – Prostate, Lung, Colon and Ovary [9]

76 000 + men (aged 55–74 years) enrolled in multi-centre trial in the USA

Randomly assigned to intervention (organised annual PSA testing for 6 years and annual DRE for 4 years) vs. Control (usual care including opportunistic screening

No difference in PCa mortality in organised systematic annual PSA testing vs. opportunistic PSA testing (although 52% of control arm had ad hoc screening)

ProtecT Trial (2017) – PROstate Testing for Cancer and Treatment [10]

Obtained men from "PCa study" – 82,000 recruited (aged 50–69 years) between 1999 and 2009 via PSA test, of which 2664 received diagnosis of localised PCa.

Patients then randomised equally between Radiotherapy (RTx) vs. Radical Prostatectomy (RP) vs. Active Surveillance (AS)

Primary outcome – PCa mortality at 10 years follow up

No significant difference was found between treatment modalities.

ERSPC Study (2013) – European Randomised study of Screening for Prostate Cancer [11]

Multi-national European study group, publish their ongoing results of meta-analysis of RCTs.

Screening arm vs. Observation arm

Latest with 13 year median follow up: NNT is 27 (27 PSA screens would have to be treated to prevent 1 death) and 781 PSA screens to avert 1 death.

PSA screening reduced cancer-specific death rates by 20%, no difference in OS.

PATHOLOGY

>95% of PCa arises from the prostatic acinar or ductal epithelium (adenocarcinoma).

The critical feature in prostate adenocarcinoma is *absence of the basal cell layer* (including absence of staining for basal cell markers p63 and cytokeratin 34BE12).

The basement membrane is breached by malignant cells (small glandular acini) which invade into prostatic fibromuscular stroma.

75% of cases originate in peripheral zone – more frequently associated with extra-capsular extension, seminal vesicle extension, lymph node (LN) metastases.

20% in transitional zone – arise near foci of BPH and are usually smaller in size and better differentiated at cellular level.

5% arise in embryologically distinct central zone.

Prostatic sarcomas – rare, mainly in childhood, usually as rhabdomyosarcoma

Local spread is often along course of autonomic nerves (peri-neural invasion). Rarely does PCa extend beyond Denonvillier's fascia into the rectum.

Bony metastases are characteristically *sclerotic* (rarely lytic) – most commonly occur in axial skeleton (ribs, spine, pelvis) followed by proximal long bones, skull.

Lymph nodal spread – most commonly to obturator fossae, iliac (common / internal / external)

HIGH GRADE PROSTATIC INTRA-EPITHELIAL NEOPLASIA

Consists of architecturally benign prostatic acini and ducts lined by cytologically atypical cells.

The basal cell layer is present although basement membrane may be fragmented.

High vs. Low- grade depending on prominence of the nucleoli.

HGPIN is a proposed precursor to PCa but definitive evidence of this remains unproven. The site of HGPIN does not correlate with future site of detection of PCa.

Exists in 4 grades (tufting, micro papillary, cribiform, flat) however 97% are tufting and there are no known clinically relevant differences between the different architectural patterns.

HGPIN does not secrete PSA. [13]

If 1 biopsy core features PIN – chance of PCa on repeat biopsy is 20% (ie. do not repeat biopsy), if > 1 core – chance can be 70%.

EAU recommend repeat biopsy if 3+ cores contain HGPIN (time interval undefined). [14]

ATYPICAL SMALL ACINAR PROLIFERATION

Acini are lined with cytologically abnormal epithelial cells and may exhibit atrophic features. Basal layer is focally absent, columnar cells have prominent nuclei.

Has a higher detection of PCa on repeat biopsy (40%) than HGPIN, therefore the EAU guidelines recommend repeat biopsy (time interval undefined). [14]

However the rate of Gleason 7+ cancers on subsequent biopsies is very low, so patients with ASAP could alternatively be managed with PSA surveillance alone. [15]

OTHER PROSTATE CANCER SUB-TYPES

Intra-ductal (0.5% of cases) arising from prostate ducts, typically aggressive (Gleason 8 or more)

Mucinous adenocarcinoma is rare, aggressive, associated with early metastases, high PSA + ALP.

Small cell carcinoma (occasionally secretes ADH, ACTH), leiomyosarcoma (mesenchymal tumour)

GLEASON GRADING

Developed in 1966 by pathologist Donald Gleason.

Adenocarcinoma is graded 1–5 according to its gland forming differentiation. [Table 2]

2–6 (well differentiated), 7 (moderately differentiated) and 8–10 (poorly differentiated)

Table 2 – Gleason grading system for prostate cancer

Grade 1	Well-demarcated nodule
Grade 2	Irregular spacing between glands and irregular outline
Grade 3	Variability in gland shape and spacing
Grade 4	Gland fusion
Grade 5	Diffuse solid sheet of undifferentiated cells

The scoring process:
- 2 most dominant types added to give score

- if only 1 pattern is observed, double the grade to give the score
- if 3 grades observed, score the most common plus highest grade (irrespective of extent)
- if predominantly G4 / 5, do not incorporate G3 if this is < 5%

Gleason scoring correlates well with prognosis and crude survival, significant predictor of time to recurrence after RP.

Most important prognostic indicator following radical treatment. [17]

Good inter-observer reproducibility. However the scoring can be affected by RTx and 5ARIs (to exhibit score 8–10) and as such pathologist may not wish to report.

Cytological features do not play a part in Gleason grading.

Under-estimation of score is more common (30–40% after RP specimens are analysed) whilst over-estimation is uncommon. (5%)

INTERNATIONAL SOCIETY OF UROLOGICAL PATHOLOGY (2014)

ISUP modified the Gleason score of biopsy detected PCa to align PCa grading with other cancers and to further qualify the highly significant distinction between G3+4 and G4+3. [18] [Table 3]

Table 3 – ISUP grading of biopsy proven prostate cancer

Gleason Score	ISUP Grade	
2–6	1	
7 (3 + 4)	2	
7 (4 + 3)	3	Consider full staging scans at diagnosis
8 (4 + 4) or (5+3) or (3 + 5)	4	(i.e. bone scan and CT TAP)
9–10	5	

PROSTATE SPECIFIC ANTIGEN (PSA)

PSA is a 34kD serine protease, an organ-specific (not cancer-specific) glycoprotein, and is produced by the columnar acinar and ductal prostatic epithelial cells.

Encoded on chromosome 19.

PSA also known as hk3 (member of kallikrein family) and its function is to liquefy the seminal coagulum within the ejaculate to facilitate fertilisation.

PSA exists in 3 forms within serum:

1. *Unbound* (half-life 2 hours) – small fraction of total [cleared by kidney]
2. (Majority) *bound to ACT* – (half life 4 days) [cleared by liver]
3. *Bound to AMG* (half life 4 days) – not used for measuring purposes

PCa patients have a greater fraction of PSA complexed to ACT (i.e. lower free PSA in PCa). [19]

Overall PSA half-life is 2–3 days.

PSA is a million times more concentrated in semen compared to serum.

1g BPH produces 0.15–0.3 ng / ml of PSA.

5ARIs will lower PSA levels by 50% after 6 months of treatment, however the ratio of free to bound PSA remains unchanged. [20]

Cancer cells produce less PSA (mRNA and protein) than normal prostate or BPH cells. The reason for PSA elevation in cancer (and inflammation) is architectural glandular disruption.

In benign epithelium PSA is intensely expressed compared to hK2, in contrast to cancerous tissue in which more intense expression of hK2 is seen.

PSA measurement: Total PSA = Free PSA + Complexed PSA (only ACT bound)

There is no absolute cut-off PSA below which prostate cancer cannot be present.

Table 4 – Oesterling age-specific reference ranges for PSA [21]

Age	PSA (ng/ml)
40–49	2.5
50–59	3.5
60–69	4.5
70–79	6.5

80% of men with PCa and PSA < 4 have organ confined disease.

66% of men with PCa and PSA 4–10 have organ confined disease.

>50% of men with PCa and PSA > 10 have disease beyond the prostate.

Consider using the ERSPC risk calculator for PCa (based on PSA, prostate volume, age etc.).

PSA VELOCITY

Defined as the rise in PSA per year (in ng/ml/year).

PSAV should be calculated with at least 3 separate PSAs, and a rise of > 0.6–0.75 ng / ml / year in PSA is associated with increased risk of PCa. [22]

PSAV = 0.5 x ((PSA 2 – PSA 1/ time 1 in years) + (PSA 3 – PSA 2/ time 2 in years))

PSA DOUBLING-TIME

Defined as length of time for PSA to double in months or years (calculated using regression analysis of recorded PSA tests).

PSADT can help in patients with high PSA but negative biopsy, monitoring low-risk disease, or rising PSA following radical treatment. [23]

PSA DENSITY

Defined by the serum PSA per millilitre of prostate tissue (PSA / Volume in ml). [24]

Prostate volume (ellipsoid formula) = height x width x length x 0.52

Normal is < 0.15 ng/mL^2. Difficult to quantify volume of prostate.

Alternatively use PSATZD (amount of PSA / mL of transitional zone tissue).

FREE TO TOTAL PSA

Defined as ratio of free PSA to total serum PSA. [25]

In BPH the f/T PSA ratio is significantly higher, however this is not currently used as diagnostic test for PCa.

SUPER-SENSITIVE PSA

Allows PSA to be detected to a threshold of 0.003 ng / ml.

Potential application for the early detection of biochemical relapse after RP. [26]

UPM3 TEST

Detects prostate cancer antigen 3 (PCA3) which is a gene produced by prostate epithelial cells 60–100 times more in PCa vs. Benign disease. [27]

Collect first 20ml of urine after prostatic massage for analysis.

STAGING [1]

Table 5 – TNM staging for prostate cancer

T – Primary Tumour	
TX	Primary tumour cannot be assessed
T0	No evidence of primary tumour
T1	Clinically inapparent tumour that is non-palpable
	T1a – Tumour incidental histological finding in ≤ 5% of tissue resected
	T1b – Tumour incidental histological finding in ≥ 5% of tissue resected
	T1c – Tumour identified by needle biopsy (e.g. patient with elevated PSA)
T2	*Tumour that is palpable and confined within the prostate*
	T2a – Tumour involves one half of one lobe or less
	T2b – Tumour involves more than half of one lobe, but not both lobes
	T2c – Tumour involves both lobes
T3	*Tumour extends through the prostatic capsule*
	T3a – Extracapsular extension (unilateral or bilateral) including microscopic bladder neck involvement
	T3b – Tumour invades seminal vesicle(s)
T4	Tumour is fixed or invades adjacent structures other than seminal vesicles: external sphincter, rectum, levator muscles, and/or pelvic wall
N – Regional Lymph Nodes	
NX	Regional lymph nodes cannot be assessed
N0	No regional lymph node metastasis
N1	Regional lymph node metastasis (regional include true pelvic nodes i.e. pelvic nodes below the bifurcation of common iliac arteries)

M – Distant Metastasis	
M0	No distant metastasis
M1	Distant metastasis
	M1a Non-regional lymph node(s)
	M1b Bone(s)
	M1c Other site(s)

N-STAGING

Pelvic lymphadenectomy is the gold-standard assessment of N-stage in PCa. [28]

This should be undertaken bilaterally even if prostate biopsy is positive unilaterally (contra-lateral LN involvement in 1/3 cases).

Low risk patients (predicted risk < 10%) should be spared from pelvic lymphadenectomy.

PSA alone is unhelpful for predicting LN metastasis.

CT and MRI have low sensitivity and specificity – as microscopic LN invasion does not enlarge nodes, and size of non-metastatic LNs vary and overlap with size of metastatic nodes. [29]

Choline PET / CT

11C or 18F choline PET can be used as alternative for LN assessment, however sensitivity and specificity do not match pelvic lymphadenectomy. [30]

Roach formula – 2 / 3 PSA + (10 x [Gleason – 6]) = % likelihood of LN mets

Partin's Tables

Use Gleason score, PSA, clinical PCa stage – to predict risk of seminal vesicle involvement, extra-capsular extension, lymph nodal involvement. [31]

Derived from RP specimens (EPLND rarely performed so nomograms prone to under-estimation).

M-STAGING

Tc-99m bone scan is most widely used imaging technique for detecting bony metastases in PCa.

Sensitivity and specificity approximately 80%.

MDP is taken up by areas of bone with increased blood supply and osteoblastic activity.

Confounding lesions include old fractures, osteomyelitis, TB, benign bone lesions (eg. osteoma).

Independent predictors of bone scan positivity include PSA, Gleason score and clinical stage. [32]

PSA 20–50 will feature positive bone scan in 16%.

PSA 10–20 will feature positive bone scan in 5%.

18F-sodium fluoride PET has highest sensitivity for detecting metastases, but is less cost-effective. It does not detect LN metastases as well as choline PET does.

Whole body MRI is more sensitive and specific than bone scan or CT.

Choline PET has higher specificity for metastases than Tc-99m bone scan.

MRI IN PCA

Requires 1.5 or 3 Tesla scanner, a dedicated uro-radiologist, multi-parametric (T2-weighting, diffusion weighting, dynamic contrast enhancement)

T2-weighted imaging remains the most useful method for local staging on mpMRI.

T2 – water is bright (peripheral zone bright as high water content) and PCa will appear as low signal abnormality on MRI.

False negative rate 5–25%

Endo-rectal MRI appears more accurate for T-staging compared to surface MRI [33] however patients find this uncomfortable and it has not gained wide acceptance.

DW-MRI relies on Brownian motion of water molecules. In areas with densely packed tumour cells, diffusion of the molecules is impeded (i.e. restricted diffusion) and thus appear bright.

DCE imaging relies on fast T1 images after gadolinium contrast, to assess tumour angiogenesis (rapid wash in / wash out).

PROMIS Study [34] (PROstate Mri Imaging Study)

Multi-centre study published in 2017.

Inclusion criteria: PSA < 15, no previous biopsy (n = 576 patients)

All patients underwent mpMRI, TRUS and template biopsy. Conduct of tests all blinded to other results. Clinically significant PCa defined as Gleason 4+3 or above.

MRI could detect higher-risk disease with greater sensitivity than TRUS biopsy. Allowed greater detection of clinically significant PCa in conjunction with biopsy.

mpMRI when added to TRUS diagnosed 18% more cases than TRUS alone.

NPV of mpMRI was 89% and could have avoided 1 in 4 biopsies.

mpMRI sensitivity 93%, TRUS sensitivity 48%

PIRADS Scoring

Standardised system of reporting level of suspicion the reporting radiologist has for presence of a clinically significant PCa on MRI [35]

Table 6 – PIRADS scoring system for prostate cancer

PIRADS 1	Highly unlikely
PIRADS 2	Unlikely
PIRADS 3	Equivocal
PIRADS 4	Likely
PIRADS 5	Highly likely

PRECISION Study

Multi-centre randomised trial of 500 men with clinical suspicion of PCa, no previous biopsy

Assigned to TRUS vs. MRI + targeted TRUS (if MRI was suspicious, TRUS was then performed).

Outcome – more clinically significant PCA found in MRI+TRUS group compared to TRUS alone.

PROSTATE BIOPSY

Performed with 7.5 MHz trans-rectal US probe and 18G Trucut biopsy needle.

Indications for performing a TRUS biopsy:
- abnormal DRE and / or elevated PSA
- previous biopsy showing multi-focal PIN or ASAP
- previous negative biopsy but rising PSA and / or abnormal DRE
- part of active surveillance protocol for low-risk disease

TRUS is not superior to DRE in detecting organ-confined PCa.

Risk of severe sepsis (1–2%) [36] – give IV gentamicin, PR metronidazole, PO quinolone.

Obtain informed consent – risks of sepsis, bleeding, urinary retention, pain. Perform DRE. Measure prostate volume using ellipsoid formula.

12 cores accepted compromise – length of biopsy significantly correlates with PCa detection.

Use 10mL of 2% lignocaine using long spinal needle.

The *Vienna nomogram* is a tool to guide number of cores to be taken, taking into account age and prostate volume in mL. [37]

If PSA 4–10 ng / mL and patient has negative TRUS biopsy, the chance of positive second biopsy (22%) or third (10%).

Hypo-echoic lesions include granulomatous prostatitis, BPH nodules, PCa, however haematological malignancies are *iso-echoic*.

Corpora amylacea are calcifications most commonly seen between transitional and peripheral zones of prostate.
- diffuse calcifications across prostate occur naturally with age
- large calcifications could be calculi which may be relevant in context of infection

The finding of peri-neural invasion on biopsy suggests higher risk of capsular penetration. [38]

Peri-neural invasion in radical prostatectomy specimens has no prognostic value.

TEMPLATE-GUIDED SATURATION BIOPSY

Template biopsy is performed under GA with 30–50 cores, targeted biopsy involves fewer cores. Similar risks to TRUS biopsy – higher risk of urinary retention (5%).

Template biopsy enhances the identification of transition zone cancers not detected by previous TRUS biopsy in patients at high risk of PCa. [39]

RISK STRATIFICATION

Establishing a patient's risk group allows you to determine the most appropriate staging investigations and treatment.

Table 7 – NICE Guidelines (2014) risk category assignment for localised PCa [40]

Level of risk	PSA		Gleason score		Clinical stage
Low risk	< 10 ng/ml	and	≤6	and	T1–T2a
Intermediate risk	10–20 ng/ml	or	7	or	T2b
High risk[1]	> 20 ng/ml	or	8–10	or	≥T2c
(Locally advanced)	Any PSA		Any (Any ISUP)		cT3–4 or N⁺

1 – High-risk localised prostate cancer is also included in the definition of locally advanced prostate cancer

TREATMENT

Table 8 – Treatment options recommended by NICE guidelines [40] according to risk group:

	Low Risk	Intermediate Risk	High Risk
Watchful waiting	Option	Option	Option
Active surveillance	Preferred	Option	Not recommended
RP	Option	Preferred	Preferred
Brachytherapy	Option	Option	Not recommended
Conformal RTx	Option	Preferred	Preferred
Cryotherapy	Not recommended	Not recommended	Not recommended
HIFU	Not recommended	Not recommended	Not recommended

WATCHFUL WAITING

Defined as the conscious decision to avoid treatment until required when symptoms of progressive disease develop.

Criteria for selecting WW as management strategy:
- life expectancy < 10–15 years
- significant co-morbidities which preclude radical treatment
- low-grade or low stage PCa

Charlson Co-morbidity Index is method of predicting mortality by classifying co-morbidities. [41]
- A score of 2+ implies patient will most likely die from other causes by 10 years follow up
- Check the CCI before proceeding to TRUS biopsy

The 10-year cancer specific mortality for WW patients is 15% and risk of metastases is 20%.

ACTIVE SURVEILLANCE

Management option for men who have potentially curable PCa but wish to avoid the complications associated with intervention.

The aim is to avoid treatment in those men with indolent cancers by only treating those with signs of progression (AS may avoid radical intervention in 60–80% of patients).

The Royal Marsden Criteria for selecting AS: [42]

- age 50–80
- fit for radical treatment
- PSA < 15 ng / ml
- Stage T1 / 2
- Gleason 3+4 or less
- < 50% positive cores

NICE recommend AS for all men (above 50 years) with low-risk disease who would be fit for radical treatment. Lack of consensus about optimal follow up regime.

The follow up for patients on AS according to NICE:

- DRE is performed at least once a year
- PSA every 3 months for one year, 6-monthly thereafter (monitor PSA kinetics throughout)
- mpMRI prior to entry into AS
- repeat TRUS biopsy after 12 months, but not routinely thereafter
- consider repeat MRI or TRUS if clinical scenario changes

Switching to active treatment should be considered:

- upon patient request
- change in T-stage on mpMRI
- change in biopsy: Gleason score, number of involved cores, length core involvement
- PSADT < 2 years (less powerful indicator)

Canadian study by Klotz (2005) of 450 low-risk AS patients – a third came off AS, at 8 years the cancer specific survival was 99%. [43]

Table 9 – Summary of the differences between AS and WW

	Watchful Waiting	Active Surveillance
Aim	Avoid treatment	Treat only if necessary
Protocol	Occasional PSA, no biopsies	Frequent PSA, repeat biopsy
Treatment indication	Symptoms	PSADT, Biopsy change
Treatment timing	Late	Early
Treatment intent	Palliative	Curative

RADICAL PROSTATECTOMY (RP)

RP may be performed open, laparoscopic or robot-assisted. The functional and oncological outcomes are comparable.

Patient >10-year life expectancy pre-operatively is paramount.

EAU Guidelines recommend all approaches are acceptable.

Laparoscopic and robotic are associated with less bleeding vs. open (due to pneumoperitoneum).

The most common site of positive margins on RP specimen is at the apex.

Complications include:
- Early – bleeding (5%), infection (5%), mortality (<1%), rectal injury (5%)
- Late – impotence (40–60%), stricture / stenosis (10%), incontinence (below)

Incontinence mild in 50% at one year, 5% severe long term which may benefit from intervention after 12 months: bulking agents, sling or AUS (only surgery recommended by NICE).
- Patients should be taught PFEs prior to surgery

Impotence can be treated with PDEi (pre-op or early post-op as penile rehabilitation).

Contra-indications to NS surgery include:
- palpable disease (if unilateral can preserve other side)
- high Gleason score
- high chance of capsular breach

Unilateral NS (50% potent), bilateral NS (60% potent)

Neuro-vascular bundles are located in lateral pelvic fascia between prostatic and levator fasciae.

Nerve-sparing RP can be undertaken in most men with localised PCa (not if T2c / T3 i.e. risk of extra-capsular extension) or high-risk factors (e.g. Gleason > 7 on biopsy, very high PSA).

Preservation of seminal vesicles does not improve potency, incontinence or margin status.

Preservation of bladder neck does not improve potency, continence, strictures or margin status.

Extra-peritoneal approach avoids bowel manipulation, no difference on margin status.

The 10-year survival figures following RP are:

- OS (>95%), metastasis free (90%), PSA free (70%)

Therefore almost 1 in 3 patients experience PSA failure after RP, the majority within first 3 years.

Biochemical recurrence after RP is defined as 2 PSA readings > 0.2ng / mL and rising.

PIVOT (Prostate cancer Intervention Versus Observation Trial) [44]
- USA study comparing WW vs. RP
- no overall survival (OS) or cancer specific survival (CSS) between two arms
- sub-group analysis showed benefit of RP in intermediate and high-risk disease

SPCG-4 (Scandinavian PCa Group) [45]
- compared WW vs. RP for (T2 or less PCa) (low and intermediate risk)
- 695 patients analysed
- higher CSS in RP group < 65 years of age

Low-Risk PCa

The decision to offer RP in low-risk PCa should be based on probability of clinical progression, side effects and potential benefit to survival.

Pelvic LND is not necessary as the risk for node positive disease is < 5%.

Intermediate-risk Localised PCa

SPCG-4 suggested significant reduction in death from PCa and metastases when comparing WW vs. RP in intermediate-risk disease. [45]

PIVOT showed reduced all cause mortality but not death from PCa (subgroup analysis). [44]

Positive LN risk is 4–20% therefore EPLND should be offered only if risk is perceived >5%.

High-risk + Locally Advanced PCa

Patients are at increased risk of PSA failure, metastatic progression, PCa death.

There is no consensus regarding optimal treatment for men with high-risk PCa. EPLND should be performed in all patients (positive LNs 15–40%) and tumour must be low volume, not invading sphincter or fixed to pelvic wall.

Pelvic LN Dissection

EPLND during RP does not improve oncological outcomes.

Provides staging / prognostic information not matched by any other available procedure.

"Briganti nomogram" [46] or "Roach Formula" [47] are tools to assess risk of LN positive disease.

Frozen section LN analysis should no longer be performed.

Adjuvant Treatment

Do not offer adjuvant hormonal therapy after RP for pN0 disease.

If pT3 N0 with high risk of local failure (positive margins, capsular rupture, seminal vesicle invasion), salvage RTx may be offered.

Alternatively monitor PSA and offer salvage RTx once PSA > 0.5 ng / mL.

If pN1 disease noted then offer early adjuvant androgen ablation therapy (10 year CSS of 80%), with or without adjuvant RTx (optimal field remains unclear).

Neo-adjuvant Treatment

Hormone treatment prior to RP has been shown to reduce prostate volume and positive surgical margin rate, however no evidence of improved CSS and therefore not recommended.

RADICAL RADIOTHERAPY

RTx is the use of ionising radiation to achieve fatal damage to neoplastic cells.

In external beam RTx, X-rays (photons) are produced by a linear accelerator which accelerates electrons abruptly stopping them with a metal target (kinetic energy converted into X-rays).

The energies required to generate XRs capable of penetrating human tissue are in Megavoltage range (typically > 8MV).

The inverse square law of electromagnetic radiation states that as distance from radiation source doubles, the intensity falls to one quarter (principle exploited by brachytherapy).

RTx works by a proportion of the XR energy being absorbed by proliferating tissues, generating free radicals which result in DNA damage and irreparable double-strand breakage.

Radiobiology promotes the "four R's" of the radiation response:

Repair – DNA repair occurs after RTx, cells are more radio-sensitive in G2 or S phase of cell division, fractionation allows more cells to be in sensitive phase.

Reoxygenation – O_2 required for free radical formation, as more cells die then more O_2 becomes available.

Reassortment – cells in G0 (rest) phase will not express damage immediately until cell division occurs, however G2 + S phase are radiosensitive, so ideally RTx should be given to catch the opportune moment of cell division.

Repopulation – viable tumour cells continue to divide, which compromises efficacy.

The energy absorbed is measured in Gray (1J of energy per kg of tissue = 1Gy)

NICE states minimum dose of 74Gy should be delivered to prostate (no more than 2Gy per visit).

Intensity Modulated Radiotherapy (IMRT) – is a newer technique using computer technology to modify intensity + shape of RTx to match prostate shape/size (allows greater Gy dosage).

Linear quadratic Model

Uses two co-efficients alpha (A) and beta (B) to describe dose response relationship. A is probability lethal damage by single event (e.g. ds-DNA break), B is by two separate events.

The A/B ratio of a tissue will determine how it behaves to changes in fractionation.

Early responding tissues (skin, marrow and tumour) are triggered to respond and proliferate within weeks of RTx and tend to have A / B ratio (10–30Gy), the cells have little time to repair photon-induced DNA damage.

Late responding tissues (spinal cord, CNS tissue) have low cell renewal and thus good opportunity for repair between RTx fractions. The ratio here is lower (<3Gy) and thus sensitive to change in fractionation dose. (i.e. late onset of complications)

The A/B ratio for PCa is 1.5 Gy (due to its slow growth) suggesting benefit of hypo-fractionation.

CHHiP Trial (2016) – Conventional or Hypo-fractionated High-dose Intensity RTx in PCa

60 Gy in 20 fractions was non-inferior to conventional [48]

Radiotherapy Planning

Pre-treatment permanent skin tattoo is marked on the patient.

Full bladder during treatment to shift small intestine away and minimise exposed bladder tissue.

Empty rectum (by laxatives / dietary advice) to minimise size of rectum.

Contra-indications:

severe LUTS, previous pelvic irradiation, inflammatory bowel disease

Remember that most patients will have had to complete neo-adjuvant hormones prior to RTx.

Table 10 – complications after RTx for prostate cancer

Cystitis	20%
Haematuria	20%
Proctitis	30% (3% severe long term)
Urethral stricture	5%
Incontinence	1% severe long term
ED	<60% (late onset)
Second cancer	1 in 300

PSA Bounce – refers to benign rise in PSA that occurs after initial fall following RTx / BTx typically after 9 months (the PSA level should not exceed 1.5 ng / ml).

Neo-adjuvant + Adjuvant Therapy

RTx can be used in conjunction with ADT in select cases.

NICE Guidelines (2014) advise:
- neo-adjuvant hormones for 3–6 months for all patients with intermediate and high-risk localised and locally advanced PCa prior to RTx
- adjuvant hormones for 3 years post-RTx for high-risk localised + locally-advanced PCa

EORTC 22863 – [49]
- RCT (by Bolla) comparing EBRT alone vs. EBRT + 3 year of hormones (LHRH analogue)
- Disease free survival (40% vs. 74%) and OS (62% vs. 78%)
- basis of the combination of RTx + hormones which is standard practice today

Relapse Post-RTx:

Relapse post RTx is defined as any PSA increase ≥ 2ng / mL above the nadir value reached during RTx treatment.

Sequential rise in PSA can prompt investigations for recurrence such as mpMRI, PET-CT or CT.

Hormone therapy is mainstay. These do not offer further chance of cure and the time to castrate resistance is 18–24 months.

Salvage therapy is an option if there are no metastases. Salvage RP is technically challenging, salvage cryotherapy or HIFU have a potential role but lack long-term data.

Proton Beam Therapy

Proton beams are an attractive alternative to photon-beams as they deposit almost all their radiation dose at the end of the particle's path in the tissue. (Bragg Peak) with a sharp fall-off after this which minimises involvement of normal tissues.

(Bragg Peak – is a pronounced peak on the Bragg curve which plots the energy loss of ionising radiation during its travel through matter).

This is promising but currently experimental.

BRACHYTHERAPY

Involves the implantation of BTx seeds (usually 125 Iodine) under general anaesthetic in the lithotomy position.

Two stages required:
1. *Planning* (TRUS study in relation to perineal template to plan seeds) and
2. *Treatment* (60–120 seeds implanted trans-perineally) to deliver 150 Gy approx

BTx can be used as a single modality of treatment or in combination with EBRT (boost treatment).

Boost treatment has 15 year biochemical progression free survival (bPFS) of 85% (low-risk PCa), 80% (intermediate risk PCa) and 68% (high risk PCa).

NICE Guidelines advise BTx is option for PCa patients with:
- stage T2c or less
- Gleason score 7 or less
- PSA 20 ng / ml or less

Contra-indications:
- life expectancy < 5 years
- Previous TURP (high risk of incontinence)
- large prostate (>50cc) or large median lobe (difficult to implant seeds)

- coagulation disorder
- previous pelvic irradiation
- moderate to severe LUTS (risk of retention) IPSS > 12, Qmax < 15 ml/s

Complications:
- irritative LUTS, urinary retention, urinary incontinence, ED, proctitis

If local recurrence is suspected, then RP / EBRT / cryotherapy / HIFU are all options provided there are no metastases. Morbidity is greater for all these options when used secondarily.

High-dose Brachytherapy

Uses a radio-active source temporarily introduced into prostate to deliver radiation, as mono-therapy or combined with EBRT.

Note that Iridium-192 is isotope of choice.

Results are limited from very experienced centres and patients should be counselled accordingly.

Table 11 – differences between low-dose and high-dose rate brachytherapy techniques

Low-Dose Rate	Permanent seeds implanted
	I-125 used
	Dose delivered over weeks / months
	Acute side effects resolve over months
	Radiation protection issues for family
High-Dose Rate	Temporary implantation
	Ir-192 used
	Dose delivered in minutes
	Acute side effects resolve over weeks
	No radiation issues for family

CRYOTHERAPY

Uses freezing techniques to induce cell death by:
- dehydration resulting in protein denaturation

- direct rupture of cellular membranes by ice crystals
- vascular stasis / micro thrombi, resulting in ischaemic apoptosis

Done using TRUS guidance placing liquid argon or nitrogen via cryo-needles. Two freeze-thaw cycles are used at -40°C. Day case anaesthetic.

Number of cycles is the most important parameter for tissue ablation.

Frozen tissue appears hypo-echoic on US.

Potential candidates for Cryotherapy:
- low-risk or intermediate-risk PCa whose condition precludes RTx / RP
- organ confined disease
- Prostate < 40 cc

Complications – ED (up to 80%), incontinence (10%), LUTS, recto-urethral fistula

HIFU

High-Intensity Focused Ultrasound of the prostate consists of focused US waves emitted from a transducer whilst patient under GA / spinal and in lateral position.

Tissue damage achieved by mechanical, thermal (>65°C) and cavitation, and the heating causes coagulative necrosis without damaging rectal wall (maximum depth 4cm).

Patients must have low- or intermediate- risk PCa and can only have treatment in trial setting.

Complications are comparable to cryotherapy, most common is urinary retention.

Patients should be informed regarding lack of outcome data > 10 years and in the PCa salvage setting the available data is scarce.

HORMONE THERAPY

Androgen deprivation therapy (ADT) refers to any treatment that lowers androgen activity.

Prostate epithelial cells are physiologically dependent on androgens to function, grow, proliferate.

When androgen deprivation occurs, androgen-sensitive prostate cells undergo apoptosis.

Bcl-2 (anti-apoptotic protein) is normally expressed in the prostate, however over-expression is associated with development of hormone refractory disease.

p53 (facilitates apoptosis) and mutations also correlate with hormone refractory disease.

Physiology of Androgen Secretion

The hypothalamo-pituitary axis is described:
- → Hypothalamus secretes GnRH:
  - → stimulates anterior pituitary LH + FSH
    - → LH stimulates Leydig cells to make testosterone.

Testosterone is then converted to DHT (10x more active biologically) by 5-AR enzymes 1 and 2.

Once bound to the receptor in the cytoplasm, the androgen-receptor complex enters the nucleus where it interacts with DNA to influence cell growth and division.

95% of androgens are produced by the Leydig cells of testes (5% from adrenal cortex which is stimulated by ACTH).

Different Mechanisms of Inducing Androgen Deprivation

Medical and surgical forms of castration have equivalent efficacy.

Castrate serum testosterone defined as < 20 ng / dL (although in trials <50 is still used as marker)

General side-effects of ADT:
- loss of libido, ED
- weight gain, lethargy
- gynaecomastia, hot flushes, altered mood
- cognitive changes, memory loss
- osteoporosis and pathological fractures

Intermittent Hormone Therapy

IHT can be used in localised disease to limit side effects of ADT treatment, reduce the cost and preserve patient's bone density.

IHT must not cycle on / off for less than 9 months at the time as this is interval required for testosterone to restore normal levels again.

IHT is not suitable if PSA rising – currently no threshold of PSA to stop / start ADT again.

IHT aims to delay to development of castrate resistance – if ADT is stopped prior to androgen-dependent cells becoming androgen-independent, any subsequent tumour growth may remain androgen-dependent.

BILATERAL ORCHIDECTOMY

Each testis tunica albuginea is incised, seminiferous tubules excised and then defect closed.

Serum testosterone falls within 8 hours < 50 ng / dL (quickest intervention to achieve this).

LHRH AGONISTS

Synthetic long-acting analogues of GnRH given by sub-cutaneous depot injection on 1-2-3-6-12 monthly basis. e.g. goserelin acetate (brand name zoladex).

Chronic exposure and over-stimulation of the anterior pituitary by these drugs will down-regulate the GnRH receptors and thus suppress LH, FSH production and therefore testosterone.

Castrate levels are reached within 2–4 weeks.

Tumour Flare

Occurs on first administration of LHRH analogue featuring a transient surge in testosterone as the drug stimulates the anterior pituitary LHRH receptors.

Complications can include spinal cord compression, fatal cardiovascular events due to hyper-coagulation, increased bony pain, bladder outlet or ureteric obstruction.

Prevented by giving anti-androgens 1 week pre- and 2 weeks post- 1st dose of LHRH agonist.

Higher risk of occurrence in patients with high-volume disease.

LHRH ANTAGONISTS

Bind immediately to LHRH receptors leading to rapid decrease in LH, FSH and testosterone (without flare) to achieve castrate level by day 3.

Degarelix is only such drug licensed in Europe, only available as monthly depot. Definitive superiority over LHRH analogues remains to be proven.

ANTI-ANDROGENS

There are two classes of anti-androgens: *steroidal* and *non-steroidal*.

Both compete with androgens at the receptor level.

Non-steroidal anti-androgens (e.g. bicalutamide) act purely as competitors and do not affect testosterone levels i.e. preserving libido, bone density, cognition.

- gynaecomastia is common (70%)
- potential liver toxicity (must monitor LFTs)
- 150mg / day as monotherapy, 50mg / day for MAB or flare-prevention

(Gynaecomastia treated with RTx to each breast 8–10 Gy, or tamoxifen, or bilateral mastectomy)

Steroidal anti-androgens (e.g. cyproterone acetate) block androgen receptors as well as down-regulating LHRH secretion by central action.

MAB is achieved for example with zoladex + bicalutamide.

OESTROGENS

Suppress testosterone and preserve bone density.

The side effect profile and thromboembolic risk imply oestrogens not considered 1st line.

Table 12 – A summary of the different modalities of delivering ADT

Reduced androgen production	
Surgical castration	Removes Leydig cells
Medical castration	Reduces LH production
LHRH agonists	Down-regulate pituitary GnRH receptors. e.g. goserelin (zoladex)
LHRH antagonists	Inhibits GnRH receptors e.g. degarelix

Blocks androgen effect	
Non-steroidal anti-androgens	Blocks androgen at receptor level e.g. bicalutamide

Combined effect	
Oestrogen	Suppresses Leydig cells
	Inactivates androgen
	Down-Regulates LHRH secretion
Steroidal anti-androgens	Down-Regulates LHRH secretion
	Blocks androgen at receptor level e.g. cyproterone

CASTRATE-RESISTANT PCA (CRPC) TREATMENT

CRPC is defined by disease progression despite ADT and may present as serial PSA rise or development of new metastases.

EAU definition of CRPC is testosterone < 50ng / dL, and:
- radiological progression, or
- biochemical progression (3 consecutive rises in PSA one week apart resulting in x2 50% increases over nadir and PSA > 2

Androgen-independence may result from:
- development of androgen-independent clones
- over-expression of the androgen receptor
- intra-cellular synthesis of testosterone by cancer cells (targeted by abiraterone)

Treated initially with second-line hormonal therapy (maximal androgen blockade)

Third-line therapy may include cortico-steroids or oestrogens (with aspirin 75mg OD as cover).

METASTATIC PCA TREATMENT

The mainstay of treatment for mPCa is ADT (medical or surgical castration) and these are best delivered at diagnosis rather than onset of symptoms.

There is no evidence to support use of any particular modality of ADT over another (bilateral orchidectomy or LHRH antagonist are preferred in SCC presentation).

Therefore a clinically well patient presenting with mPCa could be offered:

- ADT as hormones +/- upfront docetaxel (followed by eventually MAB)
- surgical castration
- degarelix
- monitor PSA / clinical condition and potentially defer ADT in select circumstances

Clinical disease progression after ADT will occur after 12–18 months.

If PCa progresses the following options can be considered:

- 1st line: abiraterone, enzalutamide, docetaxel
- 2nd line: abiraterone, enzalutamide

Median survival of patients with newly diagnosed mPCa is 42 months.

Chemotherapy

Systemic chemotherapy is indicated in men with CRPC with proven metastatic disease (providing they have adequate renal function and good performance status).

Docetaxel up-front can increase survival by median survival by 10 months (but only 2 months if used at the time of castrate resistance). [51]

Docetaxel is given 3x weekly with prednisolone for ≤ 10 cycles.

Second-line chemotherapy agents include cabitaxel.

STAMPEDE (Systemic Therapy in Advancing or Metastatic PCa: Evaluation of Drug Efficacy) [52]

Multi-centre trial for high-risk, locally advanced or mPCa, evaluating standard of care (SOC – hormone therapy for > 2 years) plus additional medication.

2900 patients randomised between 2005 and 2013

2 (SOC) : 1 (SOC + ZA) : 1 (SOC + docetaxel) : 1 (SOC + docetaxel + ZA)

No reported significant survival benefit for (SOC + ZA) or (ZA + docetaxel)

Recommended upfront docetaxel at start of hormone therapy should become standard of care.

Abiraterone and Enzalutamide

Abiraterone acetate is CYP17 inhibitor which decreases intra-cellular testosterone level seen in castrate resistant PCa by suppressing production in cells (intra-crine) and at adrenal level.

Abiraterone must be given along with prednisolone to prevent drug-induced hyper-aldosteronism.

Enzalutamide blocks androgen-receptor transfer and compared to bicalutamide it will suppress any possible agonist-like activity.

Both are only licensed for mCRPC only.

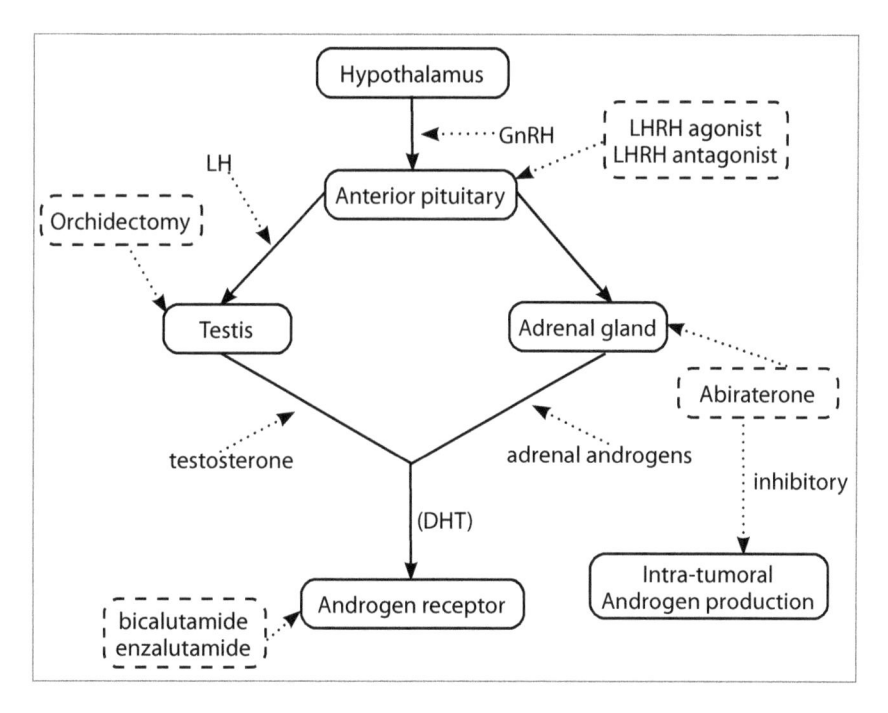

Figure 1 – Summary of different strategies of ADT for prostate cancer

mPCa Symptom Palliation

Early involvement of MDT to include palliative care, oncologist and cancer nurse specialist.

Bisphosphonates (ZA) have been shown to reduce skeletal-related events and reduce bony pain in 80% of patients with mPCa. [53]

NSAIDs are best oral option to target bone pain.

EBRT can target painful bone lesions as a single-dose.

NICE Guidelines mPCa

Offer bilateral orchidectomy to all men with mPCa as alternative to hormone therapy.

Do not offer MAB as first-line treatment.

Can offer bicalutamide mono-therapy, if sexual function preservation is priority and patient counselled regarding adverse impact on OS and gynaecomastia (if sexual function becomes unsatisfactory, stop bicalutamide and start ADT).

Offer cortico-steroid (e.g. dexamethasone) if MAB fails, as 3rd line and consider concomitant docetaxel chemotherapy.

SALVAGE TREATMENT

The timing and modality of salvage treatment after RP / RTx remain controversial.

After RP / RTx, the following salvage treatment options are available:

- salvage RTx (if previous RP) or RP (if previous RTx)
- ADT
- cryotherapy / HIFU

Observation of the patient is another option.

Although biochemical recurrence is defined as PSA > 0.2ng / mL, many advocate to wait until PSA > 0.5ng / dL before proceeding to radiological investigations (e.g. choline PET, MRI).

This is to increase the yield of positive findings.

NHS TARGET

The NHS 62-day cancer target applies to the process of prostate cancer referral, diagnosis and treatment as per the following timeline.

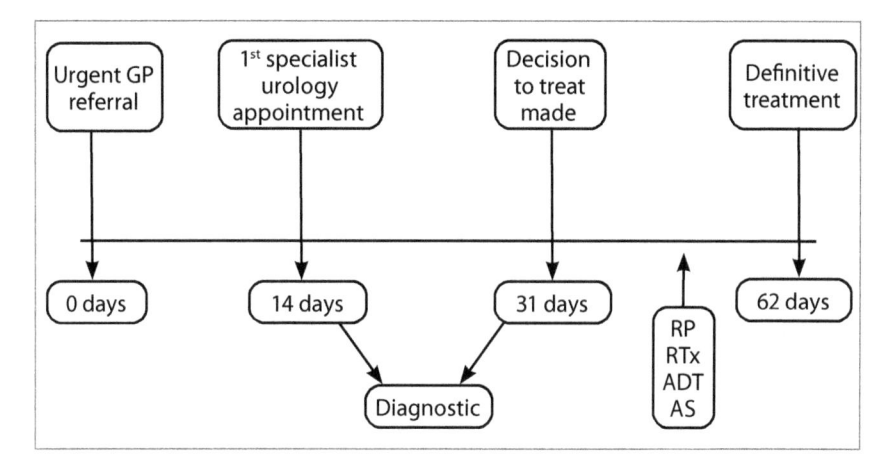

Figure 2 – NHS cancer pathway timeline for prostate cancer

TESTICULAR CANCER

EPIDEMIOLOGY

TC constitutes 1% of all male cancers, and 5% of all urological cancers. [54]

Most common solid cancer in men aged 20–45 years.

Lifetime risk is 1 in 200.

At diagnosis 1% are bilateral and >90% are germ-cell tumours.

Peak incidence for non-seminoma is 20–30 years, and 30–40 years for seminoma.

20% can present with testicular pain as their first symptom (10% of men presenting with testicular pain will have a tumour). [55]

98% of patients survive TC for ≥ 10 years in the UK.

Risk Factors

Age	if age > 60 years, more than half of men with TC will have lymphoma
	half of all TC cases occur < 35 years
	infants and young boys tend to develop yolk-sac tumours
Race	white Caucasian highest risk (also Maoris in New Zealand) > black
Previous TC	12–18x increased risk of metachronous TC
UDT	10% of TC patients have history of cryptorchidism (risk of TC 4–6x higher) [56]
	ultra-structural testicular changes by UDT occur by age 3 (ie. early orchidopexy)
	10% of developing contra-lateral TC for cryptorchidism patients
	risk of TC: 1 / 500 (normal), 1 / 125 (unilateral UDT), 1 / 45 (bilateral UDT)
HIV	increased risk of seminoma [57]
ITGCN	synonymous with CIS of the testis

	50% of cases will progress to invasive germ cell TC within 5 years
Family Hx	father (6x higher risk) and brother (8x higher risk)
Sub-fertility	poor semen analysis parameters increases risk of TC
	25% of men diagnosed with TC have oligospermia at presentation [58]

Genetic Factors

Iso-chromosome of short arm of chromosome 12 has been described in all histological types of germ cell tumours. [59]

p53 locus alterations have been identified in 66% of cases of GCNIS.

Klinefelter – (47XXY)

Kallman's syndrome – defective GnRH release (hypogonadotropic hypogonadism), most commonly presents with delayed puberty, anosmia, high risk of infertility

- mainstay of treatment is hormone replacement

PATHOLOGY

Germ cell tumours (GCTs) are a heterogenous group of neoplasms that arise mainly in gonads and rarely extra-gonadal sites along the midline (e.g. sacrum, retroperitoneum).

95% of TC are malignant GCTs – split into seminomatous (most common) and non-seminomatous both originating from germ-cells (sex cord origin & para-testicular tumours less common).

The specimen should be stored in Bouin's solution (rather than formalin) to preserve morphology.

From the pathologist's report one would require the following information:
- histological type and pathological stage
- size and multiplicity
- rete testis involvement
- presence of ITGCN
- microvascular invasion
- if seminoma, are there any non-seminomatous elements

Testicular Epidermoid Cyst

Accounts for 1% of all testicular tumours, has an onion-ring appearance on US (well-circumscribed hypo-echoic lesion with hyper-echoic margins). [60]

Not associated with ITGCN

Only perform radical orchidectomy if diagnostic uncertainty, organ preserving surgery is possible if intra-operative biopsies are negative. [61]

Table 13 – WHO classification of testicular germ cell tumours

Germ Cell Tumours	
Seminoma	
Spermatocytic seminoma (low malignant potential)	
Non-seminomatous GCT	Mature teratoma
	Teratocarcinoma
	Embryonal carcinoma
	Yolk-sac tumour
	Choriocarcinoma
Sex cord stromal tumours	
Leydig cell tumour,	
Sertoli cell tumour	Malignant, large cell calcifying, intrabular hyalinising
Granulosa cell tumour	Adult or juvenile type
Other	Mixed, gonadoblastoma
Mixed GCT / cord	
Other tumours	
Lymphoma, secondary deposits	

Seminoma

Germ cells can differentiate into spermatocytic tissue (seminoma) (40–45% of TC cases).

Seminomas have a lower metastatic potential compared to NSGCT, predominantly metastasising to the para-aortic region.

Seminomatous types of cancer are more sensitive to radiation.

Divided into classic (homogenous, lymphocytic infiltrate), spermatocytic (older men, usually benign, no ITGCN) and anaplastic (no infiltrate)

Only 10% of seminomas have raised tumour markers (always βhCG), 10% have raised LDH. [62]

Non-Seminomatous Germ Cell Tumour

Pluripotent germ cells can divide into somatic elements (teratoma) or trophoblast or yolk sac e.g. choriocarcinoma (only makes ßhCG), embryonal.

80% of NSGCTs will have raised tumour markers (60% will have raised AFP).

Leydig Cell Tumour

1–3% of TCs, 3% are bilateral, 10% are malignant.

Not associated with history of UDT.

Most commonly spreads to the retro-peritoneum – radical orchidectomy is the initial treatment, considered refractory to chemotherapy and RTx.

Tend to produce hormones and therefore create para-neoplastic syndromes: [63]
- e.g. early virilisation in children due to testosterone production
- e.g. gynaecomastia in adults due to oestrogen production

Intra-tubular Germ Cell Neoplasia (ITGCN)

Also known as TIN, is a precursor lesion for most GCTs and present in contra-lateral testis in 5% of TC patients (consider contra-lateral biopsy in all cases).

Histologically appears as malignant germ cells lining seminiferous tubules containing Sertoli cells in a single row, with nuclear pleomorphism and an intact basement membrane.
- tubules are usually of smaller diameter than normal
- show decreased / absent spermatogenesis
- atypical cells are usually aligned along the basement membrane

Overall population incidence is 0.8%.

ITGCN is the common precursor for all types of adult male GCT except spermatocytic seminoma.

- (paediatric GCTs do not typically arise from ITGCN)

ITGCN does not raise tumour markers.

Risk of progression to invasive GCT is 50% in 5 years. [64]

Increased risk for TIN includes small testis (<12 mL), history of cryptorchidism and young age. [65]

Treatment if biopsy positive for ITGCN is local RTx (16–20Gy) which causes infertility and need for testosterone replacement. Chemotherapy is less effective.

Alternative options are US surveillance or inguinal orchidectomy.

Chemotherapy can eradicate ITGCN however it is not routinely used for this purpose.

2 / 3 ITGCN patients who receive chemotherapy will have ITGCN absent on repeat biopsy, which should be repeated > 2 years after completion of chemotherapy.

Presence of ITGCN in tumour-bearing testicle does not affect the prognosis.

Choriocarcinoma

Is the only GCT which will disseminate haematogenously.

Uniformly associated with elevated hCG levels but it does not produce AFP.

These patients should always have a CT head to exclude metastases.

Caution administering chemotherapy in patients with brain metastases as these tumours are highly vascular and can bleed. [66]

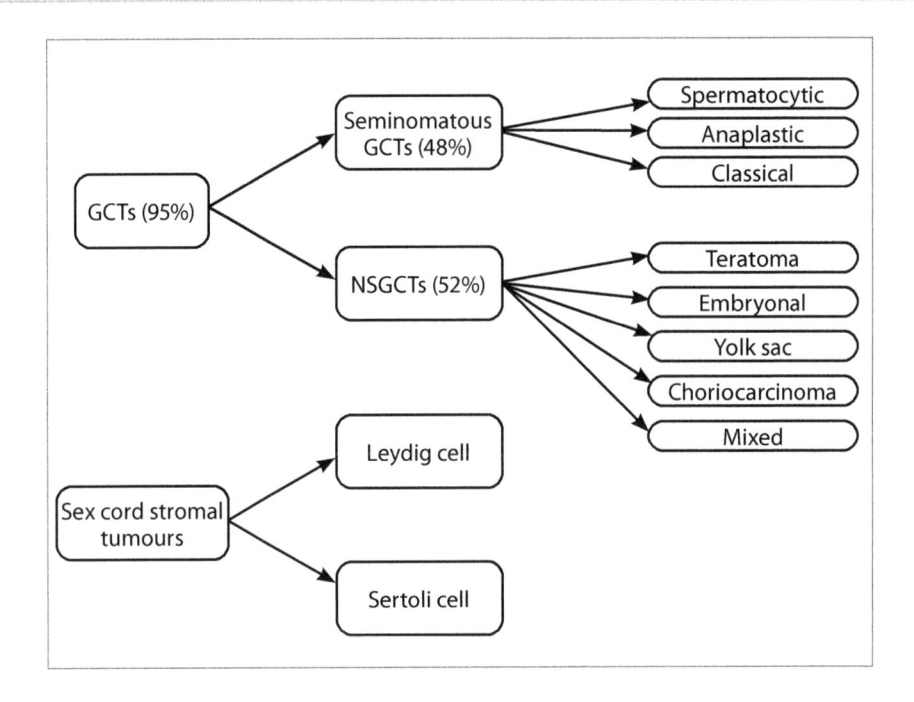

Figure 3 – Summary of pathology of different testicular tumours

TUMOUR MARKERS

Serum tumour markers are prognostic factors and contribute to diagnosis and staging.

The following should be measured before and 5–7 days after radical orchidectomy

- lactate dehydrogenase (LDH)
- alpha-fetoprotein (AFP)
- beta-HCG (βhCG)

Across the board, 50% of all TCs will have raised tumour markers, varying with the tumour type.

Presence of normal markers before orchidectomy does not exclude metastatic disease, and likewise normalisation of markers after surgery does not rule out distant disease.

90% of all NSGCTs will have a rise in tumour markers (if all measured simultaneously). [67]

Alpha-fetoprotein (Oncofetal Protein)

In 50–70% of NSGCTs there is raised AFP.

Pure seminomas do not secrete AFP – if AFP is raised in the context of seminoma this suggests a mixed element to the tumour is likely.

Serum half-life is 5 days.

Other conditions can also raise AFP – liver / pancreatic / stomach / lung malignancies and benign liver pathology

Beta-human Chorionic Gonadotrophin (Oncofetal Protein)

Expressed by syncytio-trophoblastic elements of:
- choriocarcinomas (100%)
- teratomas (40%)
- seminomas (10%)

Serum half life is 36 hours.

Other conditions can raise βhCG – liver / pancreas / stomach / lung / breast / bladder / kidney cancers and in marijuana smokers.

High levels of LH in hypo-gonadal patients can interfere with βhCG measurements and yield spuriously high readings.

Lactate Dehydrogenase (Cellular Enzyme)

Less specific marker due to elevation by other cause.

<u>Elevated in 10% of seminomas</u>, correlating to tumour burden and a useful measure of response to treatment.

Placental Alkaline Phosphatase (Cellular Enzyme)

Elevated in 40% of patients with advanced GCTs – not widely used as non-specific and can be artificially raised in smokers.

Can be histologically useful in determining the germ cell origin of a tumour.

IMAGING

US sensitivity reaches almost 100% (lesions are hypo-echoic) (7–10 MHz transducer).

These should be performed for any palpable testicular mass or retro-peritoneal mass with elevated tumour markers in the absence of palpable testicular abnormality.

Sonographic appearance of seminoma is smooth, homogenous, hypo-echoic.

Sonographic appearance of a teratoma is irregular, calcifications present and necrosis.

MRI is comparable with US for sensitivity and specificity but cost does not justify its use.

CT TAP is imaging of choice for staging.

PET has no role in the initial staging.

Testicular Microlithiasis

Features widespread calcifications throughout the testicular parenchyma and is present in 5% of the general population.

Defined as the presence of ≥ 5 calcifications (each < 2mm) per image field on US.

Incidence of TC in microlithiasis is no different to rate of population as a whole, and therefore patients can be discharged with advice to regularly self-examine. [68]

In those with significant risk factors (e.g. UDT, family history) an annual US can be considered as follow up regime along with review with urologist.

STAGING

Staging is a process by which clinically, radiologically and pathologically the extent of disease is defined to allow prognosis for relapse and survival.

The *mainstay of radiological staging is abdominal CT* (sensitivity 70% for retro-peritoneal nodes) with threshold of 3mm to define metastatic nodes.

MRI yields comparable results to CT however cost and availability are limitations, however has a role in iodine contrast-allergy, radiation reduction or poor kidney function.

American Joint Committee on Cancer (AJCC) staging classification of TNM and serum markers is shown below. The use of tumour markers in the TNM staging is unique to TC.

Table 14 – TNM staging for testicular cancer

pT – Primary Tumour	
pTX	Primary tumour cannot be assessed
pT0	No evidence of primary tumour
pTis	Intratubular germ cell neoplasia (TIN)
pT1	Tumour limited to testis and epididymis without vascular / lymphatic invasion; may invade tunica albuginea but not vaginalis
pT2	Tumour limited to testis and epididymis with vascular / lymphatic invasion; or tumour extending through tunica albuginea and vaginalis
pT3	Tumour invades spermatic cord with or without vascular / lymphatic invasion
pT4	Tumour invades scrotum with or without vascular / lymphatic invasion
N – Regional lymph nodes clinical	
NX	Regional lymph nodes cannot be assessed
N0	No regional lymph node metastasis
N1	Metastasis with a lymph node mass $\leq$ 2cm in greatest dimension or multiple lymph nodes, none > 2cm in greatest dimension
N2	Metastasis with a lymph node mass > 2cm but $\leq$ 5cm in greatest dimension, or multiple lymph nodes, any one mass > 2cm but $\leq$ 5cm in greatest dimension
N3	Metastasis with a lymph node mass > 5cm in greatest dimension
pN – Pathological	
pNX	Regional lymph nodes cannot be assessed
pN0	No regional lymph node metastasis
pN1	Metastasis with a lymph node mass $\leq$ 2cm in greatest dimension and $\leq$ 5 positive nodes, none > 2cm in greatest dimension
pN2	Metastasis with a lymph node mass > 2cm but $\leq$ 5cm in greatest dimension, or > 5 positive nodes, none > 5cm; or evidence of extra-nodal extension of tumour
pN3	Metastasis with a lymph node mass > 5cm in greatest dimension
M – Distant metastasis	
MX	Distant metastasis cannot be assessed

M0	No distant metastasis		
M1	(M1a) – distant metastasis: non regional lymph node(s) or lung		
	(M1b) – distant metastasis: other sites		

Serum tumour markers

SX	Serum markers not available		
S0	Serum markers within normal limits		

	LDH (U/l)	hCG (mIU/mL)	AFP (ng/mL)
S1	< 1.5 x N, and	< 5000, and	< 1000
S2	1.5–10 x N, or	5000–50000	1000–10000
S3	> 10 x N, or	> 50000, or	> 10000

An alternative system is the *Royal Marsden Staging System*.

- Stage 1 is disease confined to the testis
- Stage 2 includes varying degrees of retro-peritoneal nodal involvement
- Stage 3 indicates supra-diaphragmatic & visceral metastases with varying tumour markers

RADICAL ORCHIDECTOMY

This should be performed urgently on next available elective operative list (within 7 days).

Only if widespread metastasis / respiratory compromise at presentation, refer for emergency chemotherapy first and then operate subsequently.

Performed through an inguinal incision.

Prior to manipulating the testis the cord should be isolated and clamped, to allow control of draining lymphatics to minimise tumour spill.

The cord should be dissected up to the deep inguinal ring and transected. The testis, epididymis and spermatic cord are excised en-bloc.

This is curative in 75% of patients.

Tumour markers should be repeated 7 and 14 days after surgery.

The ilio-inguinal nerve is at risk of damage during the operation.

Contra-lateral Testicular Biopsy

Performed through scrotal incision, delivery of testicle and 5mm incision into tunica at each pole (double-biopsy open technique) to extrude seminiferous tubules (99% sensitivity)

- note: these must sent in Bouin's solution (not formalin)

Alternatively biopsy gun Trucut needle can be performed providing similar quality biopsy.

There is no consensus as to which patients should undergo biopsy, however recommended: [67]

- age < 40 years
- contra-lateral testicular volume < 12ml
- history of cryptorchidism
- history of sub fertility / poor spermatogenesis (Johnsen score 1–3)

ITGCN present in 5% of contra-lateral cases of TC (34% with all above risk factors).

Prostheses Insertion

Offered at the time of surgery, made of silicone and matched to size contra-lateral testis.

Complications include extrusion (5%), migration (5%), chronic pain and infection (1%). [69]

If suspected metastases (raised markers or imaging) advisable to defer prosthesis insertion as patient may need chemotherapy post-operatively which could be delayed if graft infection.

Organ-sparing Surgery

This is not routinely indicated if the contra-lateral testis is healthy.

There are certain circumstances which may warrant this: [70]

- contra-lateral TC
- single testicle (with normal testosterone levels) with tumour
- tumour volume < 30% of testicular volume
- strong suspicion of a benign tumour

TESTICULAR CANCER

Sperm Banking

EAU recommends sperm-banking prior to orchidectomy, however in practice this is difficult.

This is highly advisable if patient is known to be sub-fertile or have a small contra-lateral testis.

3 semen samples required after 3 days of abstinence.

Frozen in liquid nitrogen at -196 degrees

Screened for hepatitis B / C, HIV, syphilis

Illness at time of banking can compromise sperm quality.

Banking can occur within 7 days of chemotherapy initiation as sperm will have been produced prior to the treatment.

Chemotherapy induced azoospermia will typically have occurred within 3 months.

Cost – £200 / annum after first year, maximum storage for 10 years

STAGE 1 GCT TREATMENT

STAGE 1 SEMINOMA

Of all seminomas, 75% are confined to the testis at presentation. Only 15% will have regional nodal metastases and 10% have more advanced disease.

Following radical orchidectomy, the patient is staged and then managed by the oncologist.

Surveillance

Cure rate with orchidectomy alone is 80–85% – hence approximately 16% will relapse over a 5-year period, implying surveillance is an option. [71]

The important risk factors are: [72]

1. Tumour size > 4cm
2. Rete testis involvement

If both factors present (*high-risk*) (relapse 32%), one factor (16%) or neither (*low-risk*) (12%).

Risk-adapted approach has been developed whereby patients at higher risk of relapse are encouraged to undergo adjuvant treatment (e.g. chemo-radio therapy).

Surveillance protocols vary however one should consider:
- yearly CT of the retroperitoneum for the first 4 years after diagnosis
- 6 monthly CXR
- 3-monthly tumour marker assessment

20% of later relapses occur > 4 years, suggesting potential lifelong follow-up is required.

Adjuvant Chemotherapy

Single-dose carboplatin is the chemotherapy regime if patient wishes to have adjuvant treatment.

This has an equal efficacy to radiotherapy but is easier and quicker to deliver.

Carboplatin is much less nephrotoxic than cisplatin. [73]

Cisplatin carries a risk of ototoxicity, nephrotoxicity, sensory nerve impairment.

Adjuvant Radiotherapy

Prescribed as 20 Gy dose over 10 fractions – will reduce relapse rate to 1%.

Acute GI toxicity is common (60%) and chronic GI sequelae in 5 %.

Scrotal shield should be used to protect the contra-lateral testicle.

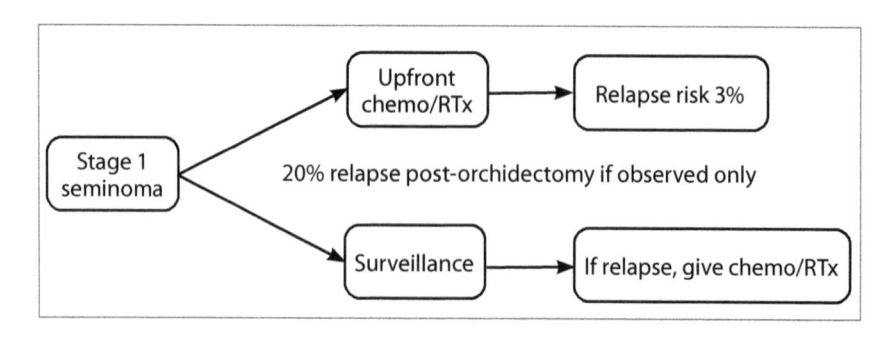

Figure 4 – Schematic approach to stage 1 seminoma management

STAGE 1 NSGCT

Following orchidectomy, the risk of relapse is higher than for seminomas.

Up to 30% of patients with CS-1 NSGCT will have sub-clinical metastases at presentation and will thus relapse during surveillance.

- (majority in lungs and retro-peritoneum)

The important risk factor is vascular invasion

- if present there is 48% risk of relapse (high-risk) and therefore chemotherapy is advised
- if absent the relapse risk is < 20 % (low-risk) and therefore surveillance is advised

Embryonal component and absence of yolk-sac component are adverse factors.

The overall survival rate bearing in mind the available treatment options is close to 100%.

Surveillance

Remains an option, however patients need careful counselling as to risks / benefits of strategy.

CT advised at 0, 3 and 12 months.

80% of recurrences will occur within 12 months.

- (1 / 3 will have normal tumour markers)

Salvage chemotherapy yields excellent survival rates > 99% hence why surveillance can be adopted with a good back-up treatment option.

Adjuvant Chemotherapy

One cycle BEP (bleomycin + etoposide + cisplatin) is recommended protocol (recent EAU update).

Poorly compliant patients may benefit from this treatment rather than surveillance CT, as would high-risk patients with vascular invasion.

One cycle of BEP does not appear to adversely affect fertility or sexual activity.

If relapse occurs after x1 BEP, then a x3 cycle is recommended.

A cycle of BEP lasts 3 weeks, consisting of 2 weeks of chemotherapy drugs, one week rest, and recommencement of the next cycle.

RPLND

In view of the high cancer-specific survival rates of surveillance, the low relapse-rate when adjuvant chemotherapy is given and excellent salvage chemotherapy option, the role of primary diagnostic RPLND has diminished.

In the UK first-line treatment is surveillance or chemotherapy.

If patient is unwilling to have surveillance or chemotherapy then RPLND can be offered.

RPLND is primarily used for de-bulking any residual tumour after chemotherapy.

RPLND in itself will diagnose 30% of patients with LN+ disease which upstages their disease to Stage II which will then require x2 BEP.

It is estimated that half the patients undergoing RPLND would not have relapsed in the first place.

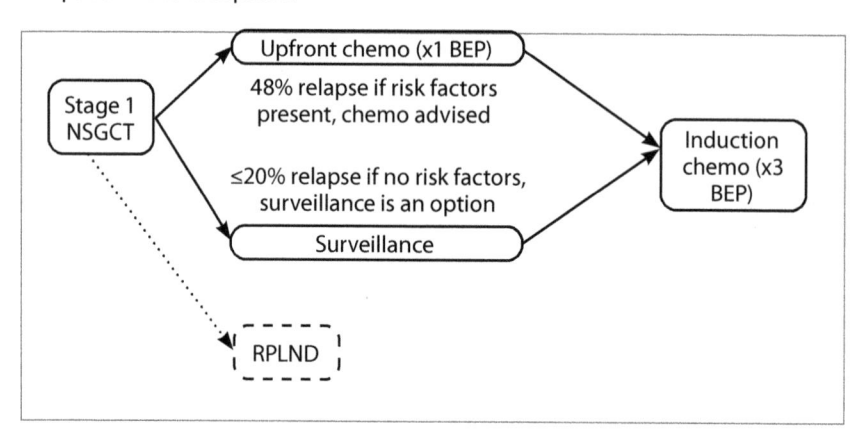

Figure 5 – Schematic approach to stage 1 NSGCT management

STAGE II A/B SEMINOMA TREATMENT

Metastatic seminomatous disease can be classified into:

- low volume disease including Stages IIA (< 2cm nodal mass) + IIB (2–5cm nodal mass)
- advanced metastatic disease including Stage IIC (nodal mass > 5cm) + Stage III (supra- diaphragmatic metastases)

RPLNs < 2cm with normal tumour markers pose a diagnostic challenge and observation for 8 weeks with repeat staging is recommended.

Chemotherapy

Mainstay UK treatment for Stage II A / B seminoma is chemotherapy (x3 BEP or x4 EP for those unsuitable for bleomycin e.g. smokers).

Chemo- and radiotherapy are equally effective. European urologists favour the use of RTx.

The major limitation of bleomycin is pulmonary toxicity.

Radiotherapy

Alternative to chemotherapy

Dosage is 30 Gy (IIA) and 36 Gy (IIB).

Distribution in IIA is further lateral compared to Stage I (to include ipsilateral iliac field) and in IIB should include an additional boost to para-aortic LNs.

STAGE II A / B NON-SEMINOMA TREATMENT

Initial chemotherapy should be given to all advanced NSGCT with raised tumour markers (except IIA with negative markers – can be managed with RPLND or surveillance).

If surveillance is chosen, repeat CT at 6 weeks and re-evaluation of size is indicated. Progression can warrant RPLND or chemotherapy.

CT- or USS- guided biopsy may be warranted as an alternative to the surveillance group.

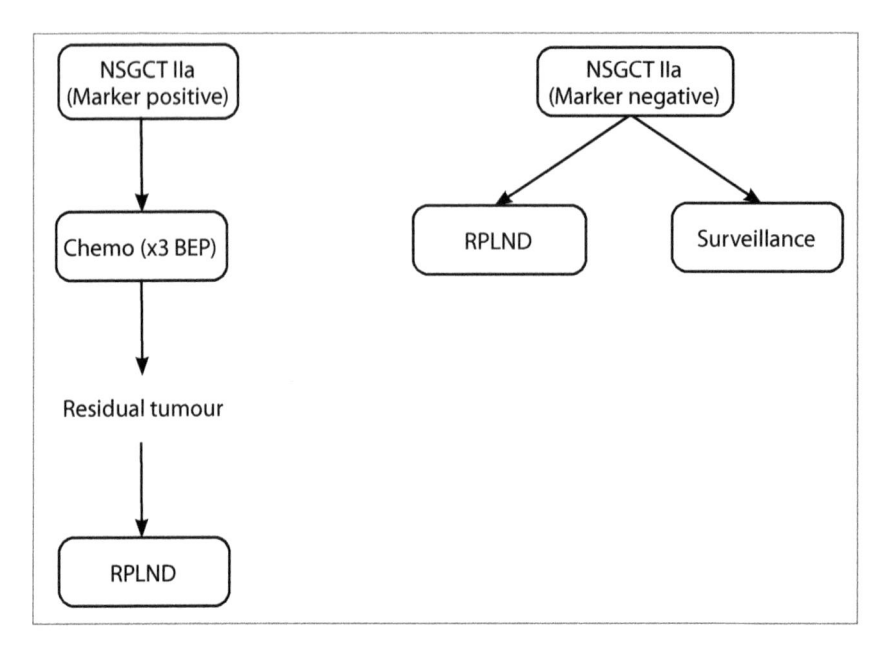

```
┌─────────────────────────────────────────────────────────────┐
│   ┌──────────────┐                      ┌──────────────┐    │
│   │  NSGCT IIa   │                      │  NSGCT IIa   │    │
│   │(Marker pos.) │                      │(Marker neg.) │    │
│   └──────┬───────┘                      └──────┬───────┘    │
│          │                              ┌──────┴──────┐     │
│          ▼                              ▼             ▼     │
│   ┌──────────────┐                ┌─────────┐  ┌──────────┐ │
│   │ Chemo (x3 BEP)│               │  RPLND  │  │Surveillance││
│   └──────┬───────┘                └─────────┘  └──────────┘ │
│          │                                                   │
│          ▼                                                   │
│   Residual tumour                                            │
│          │                                                   │
│          ▼                                                   │
│   ┌──────────────┐                                           │
│   │    RPLND     │                                           │
│   └──────────────┘                                           │
└─────────────────────────────────────────────────────────────┘
```

Figure 6 – Schematic approach to stage 2a NSGCT management

STAGE 2C / 3 (METASTATIC) TREATMENT

SEMINOMAS

Good prognosis group
- Patient should receive x3 cycles of BEP or x4 EP

Intermediate prognosis group
- Patient should receive x4 cycles of BEP

There is no poor prognosis group.

NON-SEMINOMAS.

Good prognosis group
- Patient should receive x3 cycles of BEP

Intermediate prognosis group and poor prognosis group
- Patient should receive x4 cycles of BEP

RESIDUAL TUMOUR RESECTION

Seminoma

Residual mass of seminoma should not be primarily resected irrespective of size but controlled by imaging and tumour markers.

This scenario rarely occurs and therefore tumour is not routinely expected within the mass.

PET is advised if residual volume > 3cm (4–6 weeks after chemotherapy) and if positive is a reliable predictor for viable tumour tissue in these patients.

A confirmatory biopsy is recommended.

If PET scan is positive and biopsy positive, consider RPLND.

Salvage therapy in the form of chemotherapy is given if indicated (or radiotherapy if they did not receive this initially). Surgical resection is challenging akin to retroperitoneal fibrosis.

Non-seminoma

Following first line BEP, < 10% of residual masses contain viable cancer (the vast majority harbour fibro-necrotic tissue) and salvage (second-line) chemotherapy must be considered.

This regime is PEI / TIP (cisplatin, ifosfamide and etoposide).

If residual mass is > 1cm, do not PET scan, rather refer for RPLND.

FOLLOW UP REGIMENS

Table 15 – Recommended minimal follow-up for seminoma Stage I on active surveillance or after adjuvant treatment (carboplatin or radiotherapy) [74]

Modality	Year 1	Year 2	Year 3	Year 4 and 5
Tumour markers	2 times	2 times	2 times	Once
CXR	-	-	-	-
CT / MRI	2 times	2 times	At 36 months	At 60 months

STATION 2: UROLOGICAL ONCOLOGY 2

Table 16 – recommended minimal follow-up for NSGCT Stage I on active surveillance [74]

Modality	Year 1	Year 2	Year 3	Year 4 and 5
Tumour markers	4 times	4 times	2 times	1–2 times
CXR	2 times	2 times	Once if LVI+	At 60 months* if LVI+
CT / MRI	2 times	At 24 months	At 36 months	At 60 months

Table 17 – recommended minimal follow up after adjuvant treatment or complete remission for advanced disease (excluded poor prognosis and no remission) [74]

Modality	Year 1	Year 2	Year 3	Year 4 and 5
Tumour markers	4 times	4 times	2 times	2 times
CXR	1–2 times	Once	Once	Once
CT / MRI	1–2 times	At 24 months	At 36 months	At 60 months

PROGNOSTIC TABLES

Table 18 – The International Germ Cell Cancer Collaborative Group prognostic-based staging system for metastatic seminomatous GCT [75]

Good Prognosis Group		
(90% of cases)	Normal AFP	All of the following criteria
5 – year PFS 82%	Any βhCG	Any primary site
5 – year survival 86%	Any LDH	No visceral metastases
Intermediate Prognosis Group		
(10% of cases)	Normal AFP	Any of the following criteria
5 – year PFS 67%	Any βhCG	Any primary site
5 – year survival 72%	Any LDH	Visceral metastases
Poor Prognosis Group		
No patients classified as poor prognosis group		

Table 19 – The International Germ Cell Cancer Collaborative Group prognostic-based staging system for metastatic NSGCT [75]0

Good Prognosis Group		
(56% of cases)	AFP < 1000 ng / mL	All of the following criteria
5 – year PFS 89%	βhCG < 5000 IU / L	Testis / retroperitoneal primary
5 – year survival 92%	LDH < 1.5 x ULN	No visceral metastases

Intermediate Prognosis Group		
(28% of cases)	1000 ng / mL < AFP < 10000 ng / mL, or	Any of the following criteria
5 – year PFS 41%	5000 IU / L < βhCG < 50000 IU / L, or	Mediastinal primary
5 – year survival 48%	1.5 x ULN < LDH < 10 x ULN, or	Visceral metastases

Poor Prognosis Group		
(16% of cases)	AFP > 10000 ng / mL, or	Any of the following criteria
5 – year PFS 41%	βhCG > 50000 IU / L, or	Mediastinal primary
5 – year survival 48%	LDH > 10 x ULN, or	Visceral metastases

PENILE CANCER

EPIDEMIOLOGY

> 600 new cases of penile cancer diagnosed in UK / year, < 1% of all new cancers in men in the UK and not in top 20 most common male cancers.

Incidence rates are highest in males aged > 90 years. [76]

Most cancers occur in the glans penis.

More common in developing countries where circumcision not a routine religious practice.

RISK FACTORS

Age	incidence increases as age rises
Circumcision	significantly reduces the risk (as neonatal circumcision removes half of the skin that could potentially become cancerous in the future (however adult circumcision on an otherwise healthy foreskin is unlikely to change the lifetime risk) [77]
HPV	types 16 and 18 (DNA found very commonly in intra-epithelial DNA) [78]
Phimosis	strongly associated with invasive penile cancer, due to underlying chronic infection
Smoking	confers x5 increased risk [79]
UVA	phototherapy for conditions such as psoriasis

Human Papilloma Virus

Overall 1 / 3 cases of penile SCCa show HPV infection (usually multiple strains) the most common being types 16 (70%), 6 and 18.

They are more associated with warty and basaloid SCCa.

Role as a prognostic marker is uncertain, some suggesting it has a better prognosis. [80]

PATHOLOGY

SCCa accounts for > 95% of all penile malignancies.

There are mixed forms of SCCa (warty-basaloid, verrucous) and rare types such as lymphomas or melanocytic malignancies (rare because penile skin seldom exposed to sunlight).

Secondary metastases are rare and prostatic / colorectal / bladder in origin. [81]

Is it not known how often SCCa is preceded by pre-malignant lesions.

Kaposi's sarcoma – presents with a painful raised blue / violet papule, commonly associated with HIV infection. Reticulo-endothelial tumour of penis. (Associated with herpes-virus type 8)

Most common location for penile cancer is on the glans penis.

PRE-MALIGNANT LESIONS

< 1 in 3 become malignant.

Erythroplasia of Queyrat (CIS of mucosal surface of glans or inner prepuce), a red painless circumscribed lesion which can ulcerate and bleed.

10x more likely to progress to SCCa compared to Bowen's disease.

Bowen's disease – CIS of the penile shaft or scrotal skin (does not affect glans penis which is the main difference with respect to Erythroplasia of Queyrat).

Giant condylomata – (Buschke-Lowenstein or verrucous carcinoma) aggressive locally invasive glans tumour that destroys local tissue by compression but does not metastasise.

Sporadically associated: cutaneous horn of penis, Bowenoid papulosis, BXO [82]

Carcinoma In Situ

CIS – lesion with all features of malignancy except invasion (does not cross basement membrane)

Small CIS can be treated with topical 5-FU (anti-metabolite chemotherapeutic agent that works at the S-phase causing cell cycle arrest and apoptosis) or imiquimod. [83]

Circumcision is recommended if not previously undertaken.

Benign Cutaneous Lesions

Lichen sclerosus – (BXO) commonly presents as phimosis and histologically features epithelial atrophy / thinning, loss of rete pegs, hyper-keratinisation.

Found synchronously with penile cancer in 25% of cases however direct causal links not proven.

Zoon's balanitis – red shiny erythematous patches on the glans penis

STAGING

Most commonly will start as an ulcerative / flat / papillary lesion on the glans penis (50%).

It will spread locally beneath the foreskin and then enter a vertical phase where it will invade corpora cavernosa, urethra, perineum and pelvis.

Metastasis initially to superficial inguinal LN, then deep inguinal LN, subsequently to the iliac and obturator LN.

There is no tumour marker for penile cancer.

Imaging

MRI with artificially induced erection can assess tumour invasion of the corpora as well as skip lesions. Penile MRI is highly accurate and sensitive.

USS can also evaluate corpora invasion.

Absence of palpable inguinal LN imply chance of micro-metastatic disease is 25% (however when palpable points toward metastasis as cause rather than infection).

LN can be evaluated by CT or PET-CT (highly sensitive).

A patient with palpable LN should be offered CT-TAP as part of staging.

USS along with FNA cytology will aid in confirming the diagnosis.

Penile Biopsy

Obtaining histology should address the penile lesion first, then focus on LN assessment.

In certain NHS cancer networks, Tertiary Referral Centres prefer to receive their penile cancer referrals where malignancy is strongly suspected, without prior biopsy from the referring centre.

However for the purpose of the FRCS (Urol) exam you should offer to perform a penile biopsy under (local) anaesthesia for all suspicious lesions.

Incisional biopsy – removes only part of tumour (e.g. large tumour, clearly invasive).

Excisional biopsy – removes entire lesion (e.g. if flat / plaque).

TNM Staging:

T1 category is split into two prognostically different groups, depending on presence of lympho-vascular and tumour grade (T1a and T1b).

T2 implies invasion of corpus spongiosum, while T3 implies invasion of corpora cavernosa recognising that the two invasion patters differ prognostically.

Retro-peritoneal lymph node metastases are extra-regional and therefore distant.

Table 20 – TNM classification for penile cancer [83]

T – Primary tumour	
TX	Primary tumour cannot be assessed
T0	No evidence of primary tumour
Tis	Carcinoma in situ
Ta	Non-invasive verrucous carcinoma
T1	T1a – invades sub-epithelial connective tissue without lympho-vascular invasion and not poorly differentiated (G1–2)
	T1b – invades sub-epithelial connective tissue with lympho-vascular invasion and / or poorly differentiated (G3–4)
T2	Tumour invades corpus spongiosum with or without invasion of the urethra
T3	Tumour invades corpus cavernosum with or without invasion of the urethra
T4	Tumour invades other adjacent structures
N – Lymph nodes	
NX	Regional lymph nodes cannot be assessed
N0	No palpable or visibly enlarged inguinal lymph nodes

N1	Palpable mobile unilateral inguinal lymph node
N2	Palpable mobile multiple or bilateral inguinal lymph nodes
N3	Fixed inguinal nodal mass or pelvic lymphadenopathy, unilateral or bilateral

M – Distant metastasis

M0	No distant metastasis
M1	Distant metastasis

G – Histological grading

GX	Grade of differentiation cannot be assessed
G1	Well differentiated
G2	Moderately differentiated
G3–4	Poorly differentiated / undifferentiated

pN – Lymph nodes on pathology (on biopsy or surgical excision)

pNX	Regional lymph nodes cannot be assessed
pN0	No regional lymph nodes metastasis
pN1	Metastasis in 1–2 inguinal lymph nodes
pN2	Metastasis in > 2 unilateral inguinal lymph nodes or bilateral inguinal lymph nodes
pN3	Metastasis in pelvic lymph node(s), unilateral or bilateral extra-nodal extension of regional nodal metastasis

TREATMENT

Penile preservation techniques are preferred wherever possible for functional and cosmetic outcomes, aiming however to remove the cancer completely.

Intra-operative assessment by frozen section is recommended – a margin of > 5mm is considered oncologically safe.

Penile preserving surgery has a higher local recurrence rate than radical treatment.

SUPERFICIAL NON-INVASIVE DISEASE (CIS)

Topical treatments include 5-FU or imiquimod – these should be undertaken with close surveillance and if not successful, reapplication should not be repeated.

These should not be applied in the uncircumcised male.

Imiquimod – success rate complete response > 50% (daily application for 4 weeks)

5-FU – apply 5% ointment over glans penis daily for 4 weeks, expect redness / inflammation and use condom if continuing sexual intercourse.

If using for PeIN, reassess at 6 weeks, if clear then monitor for 5 years. Do not repeat if treatment fails.

LASER ablation is an option.
- either Nd:YAG or CO2 LASER (consider aid of PDD)
- minimal sexual or urinary side effects from treatment

Total / partial glans re-surfacing
- can be primary or undertaken after failed topical therapy
- complete abrasion of glandular epithelium followed by covering with split skin graft to cover the denuded glans

TREATMENT OF INVASIVE DISEASE CONFINED TO GLANS

Circumcision – all patients should have a circumcision before considering non-surgical treatments, and this may be sufficient treatment if tumour confined to prepuce.

Glansectomy – plus reconstruction of neo-glans using split skin graft

Partial penectomy
- consent regarding: ED, penile shortening, urine spraying, cosmetic outcome
- procedure: de-glove, mobilise and ligate NV-bundle, mobilise urethra, transect penis, send frozen section, spatulate urethra, split skin graft (often from thigh), leave catheter in situ

There is no oncologically preferred penile preserving surgical technique.

Radiotherapy

No longer recommended as primary treatment option due to recurrence rate (40%).

Minimum dose 60 Gy, can boost with BTx.

Patient must be circumcised prior to RTx otherwise foreskin will fuse to glans.

Higher recurrence rate vs. Partial penectomy, salvage surgery is always an option post-RTx.

Complications include corpora cavernosa fibrosis, urethral stenosis, glans necrosis.

TREATMENT OF INVASIVE DISEASE

Confined to Glans / Corpus Spongiosum (T2)

- Total glansectomy, or partial penectomy if unfit

Invading Corpora Cavernosa and / or Urethra (T2–3)

- Partial penectomy
- Radiotherapy is an option – brachytherapy possible if < 4cm and preferable in terms of side effects, also if patient refuses surgery or is young and sexually active

T3 / T4 Disease

Total penectomy & perineal urethrostomy (with neo-adjuvant chemotherapy cisplatin-based)

Hypercalcaemia is a common complication in patients with advanced metastatic penile cancer and is due to the tumour burden rather than bony involvement (often PTH secretion).

Priapism is the most frequently encountered sign of penile metastasis.

How to perform partial penectomy:
- Cover penile lesion with condom, apply tourniquet, and make circumferential incision 1cm proximal to lesion
- Identify NVBs and ligate / divide them
- Mobilise urethra and divide
- Close corpora with 2'0 PDS in transverse fashion

SUMMARY OF SURGICAL TREATMENTS FOR PRIMARY LESION [83]

Tis / Ta / T1a – (as alternative to topical treatments or LASER), WLE with circumcision, glans resurfacing, glans resurfacing, partial glansectomy

T1b / T2 – WLE plus reconstruction, glansectomy with circumcision

T3 (minimal corporal involvement) – glansectomy and distal corporectomy

T3 (extensive corporal involvement) – partial amputation if ≥ 5cm residual stump available, if penis is small may require total penectomy

T4 – multi-modality treatment (chemo / RTx / surgery)

REGIONAL LYMPH NODE MANAGEMENT

The management of regional LN is decisive for long-term patient survival, it is curable if confined.

- Lymphadenectomy is the treatment of choice

Based on the principle that penile metastasis follows a step-wise sequence:

➜ superficial inguinal LN ➜ deep inguinal ➜ pelvic LN ➜ distant sites

Factors that increase risk of LN involvement include grade 3 disease, LVI, cavernosal involvement and sarcomatoid variants of penile cancer.

5 year survival: negative nodes (66%), inguinal nodes (28%) pelvic nodes (2%)

i.e. extent of LN metastasis is the most crucial factor in penile cancer prognosis. [84]

Involvement of regional penile MDT is recommended.

Clinically Node Negative (cN0)

Even if LN are non-palpable, 25% of patients will have micro-metastases.

Do not undertake routine CT / US for staging if LN non-palpable as these are not reliable [84] (MRI considered in select cases).

The invasive diagnostic options which are available include:

1. *Modified superficial inguinal lymphadenectomy*:
   - preserves the saphenous vein to reduce the degree of lymphoedema (20% incidence) – smaller incision and avoids transposition of sartorius muscles

- if intra-operative node positive then proceed to ipsilateral radical lymphadenectomy
- if multiple LN positive, or single LN with extra-capsular spread, then proceed to pelvic lymphadenectomy at a second operation [85]
- furthermore if 2+ positive LN are found, contra-lateral staging LN assessment should be considered

2. DSNB:
- Tc-99m injected peri-tumoral in morning, patient then goes to radiology for dynamic scanning to mark sentinel node on skin; in afternoon patient has peri-tumoral patent blue injection prior to GA, intra-operatively a gamma-ray probe detects sentinel node
- false negative 5% rate, as LN full of tumour will not uptake any radioisotope
- intra-operative use of US can reduce this rate

(Pelvic LN include distal common iliac, external iliac, obturator LN)

Both methods may still miss micro-metastatic disease.

Early lymphadenectomy is far more beneficial for long-term survival (>90%) when compared to therapeutic lymphadenectomy when nodal disease becomes palpable (<40%).

Patients must be risk-stratified:
- low-risk (pTis, pTa, or G1pT1) – could be offered surveillance (in a compliant patient)
- intermediate risk (G2T1) – surveillance / DSNB / modified lymphadenectomy
- high risk (G3, ≥ T2, LVI) – DSNB / modified lymphadenectomy

Clinically Node Positive (cN1 / cN2)

If nodes are palpable, presume metastases (estimated > 90% of palpable LN are involved with metastases) rather than infective aetiology – do not prescribe antibiotics and reassess.

Consider US + FNA along with CT TAP.

If unilateral LN are palpable with confirmed diagnosis on FNA:
- proceed to ipsilateral radical inguinal lymphadenectomy
- (if > 2 LN involved or pelvic LN or extra-capsular disease) proceed to

ipsilateral pelvic lymphadenectomy with concomitant contra-lateral DSNB / modified groin dissection (if non-palpable contra-lateral LN)

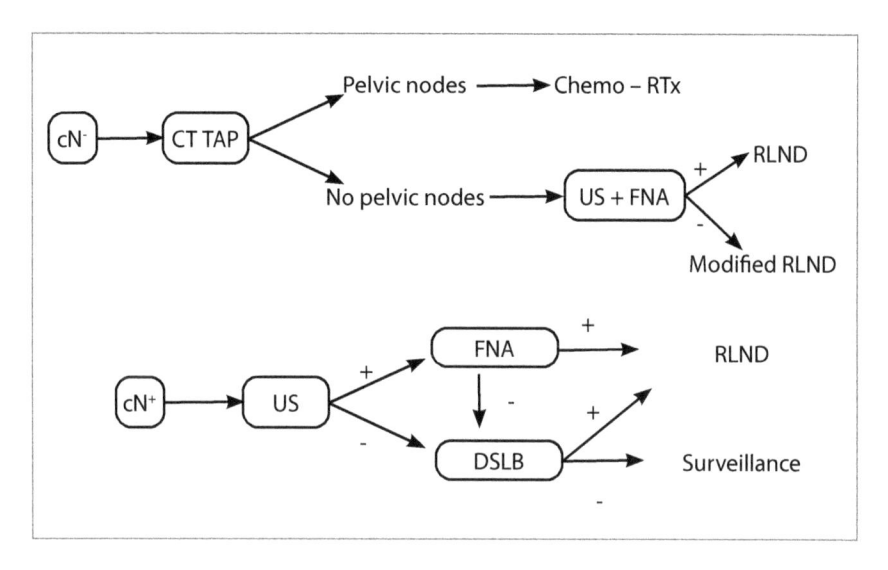

Figure 7 – Schematic approach to evaluate lymph nodes in penile cancer

Radical Inguinal Lymphadenectomy

The boundaries of the dissection are those of the femoral triangle:
- superiorly, the inguinal ligament
- laterally the lateral border of sartorius
- medially the lateral border adductor longus

Morbidity is high (50%) including infection, lymphoedema, lymphocoele. [12]

Therefore if nodes are not palpable you should not routinely subject patients to this procedure, as 75% will suffer over-treatment and high risk of morbidity.

Radiotherapy does not have an established role.

Genital Lymphoedema

Managed by mobilisation, compression stockings and underwear, scrotectomy / scrotoplasty are surgical options.

Pelvic lymphadenectomy

All sentinel nodes appear to be located inguinally – however the development of metastases will follow the route of anatomical drainage.

The next group of regional LN to become involved are the ipsilateral pelvic LN (cross-over does not occur).

CSS with pelvic LN is lower (33%) vs. inguinal only LN (70%)

Pelvic lymphadenectomy should be performed if ≥ 2 nodes are positive on DSNB. (There is no direct drainage of penile tumours to ipsilateral pelvic nodes.)

Boundaries of pelvic lymphadenectomy include:
- proximal: iliac bifurcation
- lateral: genito-femoral nerve
- medial: bladder wall
- inferior: Cloquet's node

If LN recurrence occurs after surgery, there is no consensus on treatment and this should be multi-modal with chemotherapy.

FOLLOW UP REGIMEN

Most recurrences occur within 2 years post-operatively:
- recommend follow up every 3 months for first 2 years
- 6-monthly thereafter

Follow up should include examination of penis as well as inguinal LN assessment.

URETHRAL CANCER

EPIDEMIOLOGY

Rare cancer – estimated incidence 1.5 in a million [88]

Most commonly in age > 75 years

More commonly will present with symptoms of locally advanced disease (blood discharge, bladder outlet obstruction, palpable mass, urethrocutaneous fistula.

RISK FACTORS

Exceedingly rare in those < 55 years, risk factors when TCC are similar to bladder cancer.

Infective – HPV (type 16), chronic stricture disease, sexually transmitted infections, recurrent UTIs, local radiotherapy treatment

Gender – women (x4 risk vs. men), the only urological cancer more common in females

PATHOLOGY

Occurs most commonly in bulbo-membranous urethra.

Anterior urethral carcinoma is more amenable to surgery and better prognosis than posterior urethral carcinoma.

Transitional cell carcinoma (TCC) is the most common (60%), followed by squamous cell carcinoma (20%) and rarely adenocarcinoma.

Lymphatic drainage in men will follow:

    (anterior urethra) – superficial + deep inguinal LN ➡ pelvic LN (external, obturator, internal iliac)

    (posterior urethra) – drain into pelvic LN

Lymphatic drainage in women will follow:

    (proximal 1/3) – pelvic LN chains

    (distal 2/3) – superficial + deep inguinal nodes

The WHO 1973 grading system has been replaced by the 2004 grading system, which differentiates urothelial carcinoma into papillary urothelial neoplasm of low malignant potential (PUNLMP) low-grade and high-grade.

Non-urothelial carcinoma is graded by a trinomial system (well-, moderately- and poorly-differentiated tumours).

Table 21 – Pathological grading of urethral cancer

Urothelial carcinoma	
PUNLMP	Papillary urothelial neoplasm of low malignant potential
Low grade	Well differentiated
High grade	Poorly differentiated
Non-urothelial carcinoma	
GX	Tumour grade not assessed
G1	Well differentiated
G2	Moderately differentiated
G3	Poorly differentiated

INVESTIGATIONS

Examination of the external genitalia, inguinal lymphadenopathy

Urgent cystoscopy and biopsy of the lesion

Cytology has a rather low sensitivity and should not be considered highly reliable.

Imaging – CT abdomen / pelvis / thorax. Consider MRI with artificial erection for assessment of tumour depth.

Refer for urgent discussion at regional MDT for multi-modal approach due to rarity of tumour.

STAGING

Urothelial carcinoma is classified as per table below – note that there is a separate TNM staging system for prostatic urothelial carcinoma.

Table 22 – TNM 8th edition staging for urethral cancer [89]

T – Primary tumour (urethra male and female)	
TX	Primary tumour cannot be assessed
T0	No evidence of primary tumour
Tis	Carcinoma in situ
Ta	Non-invasive papillary, polypoid or verrucous carcinoma
T1	Tumour invades subepithelial connective tissue
T2	Tumour invades any of the following: corpus songiosum, prostate, peri-urethral muscle
T3	Tumour invades any of the following: corpus cavernosum, beyond prostatic capsule, anterior vagina, bladder neck
T4	Tumour invades other adjacent organs
N – Lymph nodes	
NX	Regional lymph nodes cannot be assessed
N0	No regional lymph node metastasis
N1	Metastasis in a single lymph node
N2	Metastasis in multiple lymph nodes
M – Distant metastasis	
M0	No distant metastasis
M1	Distant metastasis

TREATMENT

Localised Primary Urethral Carcinoma

(Men) Distal tumours have better prognosis than proximal. Aim for partial urethrectomy.

Wide local excision of urethra (along with tunica albuginea) and perineal urethostomy or hypospadiac opening if length adequate.

(Women) Primary radical urethrectomy with bladder neck closure and appendico-vesicostomy.

Radiotherapy has high recurrence rates and complications.

Advanced Disease

Cisplatin-based chemotherapy – preferably neo-adjuvant before surgery rather than given alone.

REFERENCES

1. https://www.cancerresearchuk.org [last accessed 27 May 2020].
2. Kheirandish P, Chinegwundoh F. (2011) Ethnic differences in prostate cancer. British journal of cancer.105(4):481.
3. Andriole G, Bostwick D, Brawley O, et al. (2004) Chemoprevention of prostate cancer in men at high risk: rationale and design of the reduction by dutasteride of prostate cancer events (REDUCE) trial. The Journal of urology. 172(4):1314–7.
4. Lippman SM, Klein EA, Goodman PJ, et al. (2009) Effect of selenium and vitamin E on risk of prostate cancer and other cancers: the Selenium and Vitamin E Cancer Prevention Trial (SELECT). Jama. 301(1):39–51.
5. Brawer MK. (2003) Androgen supplementation and prostate cancer risk: strategies for pretherapy assessment and monitoring. Reviews in urology. 5(S1):S29.
6. Thompson IM, Ankerst DP, Chi C, et al. (2006) Assessing prostate cancer risk: results from the Prostate Cancer Prevention Trial. Journal of the National Cancer Institute. 98(8):529–34.
7. Perner S, Demichelis F, Beroukhim R, et al. (2006) TMPRSS2: ERG fusion-associated deletions provide insight into the heterogeneity of prostate cancer. Cancer research. 66(17):8337–41.
8. Andermann A, Blancquaert I, Beauchamp S, et al. (2008). Revisiting Wilson and Jungner in the genomic age: a review of screening criteria over the past 40 years. Bulletin of the World Health Organization. 86:317–9.
9. Andriole GL, Crawford ED, Grubb III RL, et al. (2012) Prostate cancer screening in the randomized Prostate, Lung, Colorectal, and Ovarian Cancer Screening Trial: mortality results after 13 years of follow-up. Journal of the National Cancer Institute.104(2):125–32.
10. Hamdy FC, Donovan JL, Lane JA, et al. (2016) 10-year outcomes after monitoring, surgery, or radiotherapy for localized prostate cancer. New England Journal of Medicine. 375(15):1415–24.
11. Ilic D, Neuberger MM, Djulbegovic M, et al. (2013) Screening for prostate cancer. Cochrane database of systematic reviews.
12. http://www.aboutcancer.com/prostate_anatomy.htm [last accessed 26 May 2020].
13. Bostwick DG, Qian J. High-grade prostatic intraepithelial neoplasia. (2004) Modern pathology 17(3):360.
14. Mottet N, Bellmunt J, Bolla M, et al. (2017) EAU – ESTRO – ESUR – SIOG Guidelines on Prostate Cancer. Eur Urol. 71(4):618–629.
15. Leone A, Rotker K, Butler C, et al. (2015) Atypical small acinar proliferation: repeat biopsy and detection of high grade prostate cancer. Prostate cancer.

16. https://orchid-cancer.org.uk/prostate-cancer [last accessed 26 May 2020]
17. Humphrey PA. (2004) Gleason grading and prognostic factors in carcinoma of the prostate. Modern pathology. 17(3):292.
18. Epstein JI, Egevad L, Amin MB, et al. (2016) The 2014 International Society of Urological Pathology (ISUP) consensus conference on Gleason grading of prostatic carcinoma. The American journal of surgical pathology. 40(2):244–52.
19. Christensson A, Björk T, Nilsson O, et al. (1993) Serum prostate specific antigen complexed to α 1-antichymotrypsin as an indicator of prostate cancer. The Journal of urology.150(1):100–5.
20. Guess HA, Gormley GJ, Stoner E, et al. (1996). The effect of finasteride on prostate specific antigen: review of available data. The Journal of urology. 155(1):3–9.
21. Oesterling JE, Jacobsen SJ, Chute CG, et al. (1993) Serum prostate-specific antigen in a community-based population of healthy men: establishment of age-specific reference ranges. JAMA. 18;270(7):860–4.
22. D'Amico AV, Chen MH, Roehl KA, et al. (2004) Preoperative PSA velocity and the risk of death from prostate cancer after radical prostatectomy. New England Journal of Medicine. 351(2):125–35.
23. Ng MK, Van As N, Thomas K, et al. (2009) Prostate-specific antigen (PSA) kinetics in untreated, localized prostate cancer: PSA velocity vs PSA doubling time. BJU international.103(7):872–6.
24. Catalona WJ, Southwick PC, Slawin KM, et al. (2000). Comparison of percent free PSA, PSA density, and age-specific PSA cutoffs for prostate cancer detection and staging. Urology. 56(2):255–60.
25. Partin AW, Catalona WJ, Southwick PC, et al. (1996) Analysis of percent free prostate-specific antigen (PSA) for prostate cancer detection: influence of total PSA, prostate volume, and age. Urology. 1;48(6):55–61.
26. Haese A, Huland E, Graefen M, et al. (1999) Supersensitive PSA-analysis after radical prostatectomy: a powerful tool to reduce the time gap between surgery and evidence of biochemical failure. Anticancer research.19(4A):2641–4.
27. Fradet Y, Saad F, Aprikian A, et al. (2004) uPM3, a new molecular urine test for the detection of prostate cancer. Urology. 1;64(2):311–5.
28. Briganti A, Blute ML, Eastham JH, et al. (2009) Pelvic lymph node dissection in prostate cancer. European urology. 1;55(6):1251–65.
29. Hövels A, Heesakkers RA, Adang EM, et al. (2008) The diagnostic accuracy of CT and MRI in the staging of pelvic lymph nodes in patients with prostate cancer: a meta-analysis. Clinical radiology. 1;63(4):387–95.
30. Husarik DB, Miralbell R, Dubs M, et al. (2008) Evaluation of [18F]-choline PET/CT for staging and restaging of prostate cancer. European journal of nuclear medicine and molecular imaging. 35(2):253–63.

31. Partin AW, Mangold LA, Lamm DM, et al (2001). Contemporary update of prostate cancer staging nomograms (Partin Tables) for the new millennium. Urology. 58(6):843–8.
32. Gleave ME, Coupland D, Drachenberg D, et al. (1996) Ability of serum prostate-specific antigen levels to predict normal bone scans in patients with newly diagnosed prostate cancer. Urology. 1;47(5):708–12.
33. Turkbey B, Merino MJ, Gallardo EC, et al. (2014) Comparison of endorectal coil and nonendorectal coil T2W and diffusion-weighted MRI at 3 Tesla for localizing prostate cancer: correlation with whole-mount histopathology. Journal of Magnetic Resonance Imaging. 39(6):1443–8.
34. Ahmed HU, Bosaily AE, Brown LC, et al. (2017) Diagnostic accuracy of multi-parametric MRI and TRUS biopsy in prostate cancer (PROMIS): a paired validating confirmatory study. The Lancet. 389(10071):815–22.
35. Hamoen EH, de Rooij M, Witjes JA, et al. (2015) Use of the Prostate Imaging Reporting and Data System (PI-RADS) for prostate cancer detection with multiparametric magnetic resonance imaging: a diagnostic meta-analysis. European urology. 67(6):1112–21.
36. Nam RK, Saskin R, Lee Y, et al. (2010) Increasing hospital admission rates for urological complications after transrectal ultrasound guided prostate biopsy. The Journal of urology. 183(3):963–9.
37. Remzi M, Fong YK, Dobrovits M, et al. (2005) The Vienna nomogram: validation of a novel biopsy strategy defining the optimal number of cores based on patient age and total prostate volume. The Journal of urology. 1;174(4):1256–61.
38. Bastacky SI, Walsh PC, Epstein JI. (1993) Relationship between perineural tumor invasion on needle biopsy and radical prostatectomy capsular penetration in clinical stage B adenocarcinoma of the prostate. The American journal of surgical pathology. 17(4):336–41.
39. Pinkstaff DM, Igel TC, Petrou SP, et al. (2005) Systematic transperineal ultrasound-guided template biopsy of the prostate: three-year experience. Urology. 65(4):735–9.
40. https://www.nice.org.uk/guidance/cg175/chapter/1-recommendations#assessment-2 [last accessed 26 May 2020]
41. Sundararajan V, Henderson T, Perry C, et al. (2004) New ICD-10 version of the Charlson comorbidity index predicted in-hospital mortality. Journal of clinical epidemiology. 57(12):1288–94.
42. van As NJ, Parker CC. (2007) Active surveillance with selective radical treatment for localized prostate cancer. The Cancer Journal. 13(5):289–94.

43. Klotz L, Zhang L, Lam A, et al. (2009) Clinical results of long-term follow-up of a large, active surveillance cohort with localized prostate cancer. Journal of Clinical Oncology. 28(1):126–31.
44. Klotz L, Zhang L, Lam A, et al. (2009) Clinical results of long-term follow-up of a large, active surveillance cohort with localized prostate cancer. Journal of Clinical Oncology. 28(1):126–31.
45. Bill-Axelson A, Holmberg L, Garmo H, et al (2014). Radical prostatectomy or watchful waiting in early prostate cancer. New England Journal of Medicine. 370(10):932–42.
46. Briganti A, Larcher A, Abdollah F, et al. (2012) Updated nomogram predicting lymph node invasion in patients with prostate cancer undergoing extended pelvic lymph node dissection: the essential importance of percentage of positive cores. European urology. 61(3):480–7.
47. Abdollah F, Cozzarini C, Suardi N, et al. (2012) Indications for pelvic nodal treatment in prostate cancer should change. Validation of the Roach formula in a large extended nodal dissection series. International Journal of Radiation Oncology* Biology* Physics. 83(2):624–9.
48. Dearnaley D, Syndikus I, Mossop H, et al. (2016) Conventional versus hypofractionated high-dose intensity-modulated radiotherapy for prostate cancer: 5-year outcomes of the randomised, non-inferiority, phase 3 CHHiP trial. The Lancet Oncology. 17(8):1047–60.
49. Bolla M, Collette L, Blank L, et al. (2002) Long-term results with immediate androgen suppression and external irradiation in patients with locally advanced prostate cancer (an EORTC study): a phase III randomised trial. The Lancet. 360(9327):103–8.
50. Ullah MI, Riche DM, Koch CA. (2014) Transdermal testosterone replacement therapy in men. Drug design, development and therapy. 8:101.
51. Tannock IF, De Wit R, Berry WR, et al. (2004) Docetaxel plus prednisone or mitoxantrone plus prednisone for advanced prostate cancer. New England Journal of Medicine. 351(15):1502–12.
52. James ND, Sydes MR, Clarke NW, et al. (2016) Addition of docetaxel, zoledronic acid, or both to first-line long-term hormone therapy in prostate cancer (STAMPEDE): survival results from an adaptive, multiarm, multistage, platform randomised controlled trial. The Lancet. 387(10024):1163–77.
53. Saad F, Gleason DM, Murray R, et al. (2004) Long-term efficacy of zoledronic acid for the prevention of skeletal complications in patients with metastatic hormone-refractory prostate cancer. Journal of the National Cancer Institute. 96(11):879–82.

54. www.cancerresearchuk.org [last accessed 26 May 2020].
55. Schottenfeld D, Warshauer ME, Sherlock S, Zauber AG, Leder M, Payne R. The epidemiology of testicular cancer in young adults. American Journal of Epidemiology. 1980;112(2):232–46.
56. Pettersson A, Richiardi L, Nordenskjold A, et al. (2007) Age at surgery for undescended testis and risk of testicular cancer. New England Journal of Medicine. 3;356(18):1835–41.
57. Frisch M, Biggar RJ, Engels EA, et al. (2001) AIDS-Cancer Match Registry Study Group. Association of cancer with AIDS-related immunosuppression in adults. JAMA. 4;285(13):1736–45.
58. Jacobsen R, Bostofte E, Engholm G, et al. (2000) Risk of testicular cancer in men with abnormal semen characteristics: cohort study. BMJ. 30;321(7264):789–92.
59. Bosl JG, Dmitrovsky E, Reuter VE, et al. (1989(Isochromosome of chromosome 12: clinically useful marker for male germ cell tumors. Journal of the National Cancer Institute. 20;81(24):1874–8.
60. Dogra VS, Gottlieb RH, Rubens DJ, et al. (2001) Testicular epidermoid cysts: sonographic features with histopathologic correlation. Journal of clinical ultrasound. 29(3):192–6.
61. Heidenreich A, Engelmann UH, Vietsch HV, et al. (1995) Organ preserving surgery in testicular epidermoid cysts. The Journal of urology. 1;153(4):1147–50.
62. Dearnaley DP, Huddart RA, Horwich A. (2001) Regular review: managing testicular cancer. BMJ. 30;322(7302):1583.
63. Al-Agha OM, Axiotis CA. (2007) An in-depth look at Leydig cell tumor of the testis. Archives of pathology & laboratory medicine. 131(2):311–7.
64. Harland SJ, Cook PA, Fossa SD, et al. (1998) Intratubular germ cell neoplasia of the contralateral testis in testicular cancer: defining a high risk group. The Journal of urology. 1;160(4):1353–7.
65. Dieckmann KP, Kulejewski M, Pichlmeier U, et al. (2007) Diagnosis of contralateral testicular intraepithelial neoplasia (TIN) in patients with testicular germ cell cancer: systematic two-site biopsies are more sensitive than a single random biopsy. European urology. 1;51(1):175–85.
66. Mandybur TI. (1977) Intracranial hemorrhage caused by metastatic tumors. Neurology. 1;27(7):650.
67. Albers P, Albrecht W, Algaba F, et al. (2011) EAU guidelines on testicular cancer: 2011 update. European urology. 1;60(2):304–19.
68. DeCastro BJ, Peterson AC, Costabile RA. (2008) A 5-year followup study of asymptomatic men with testicular microlithiasis. The Journal of urology. 1;179(4):1420–3.

69. Shukla AR, Woodard C, Carr MC, et al. (2004) Experience with testis sparing surgery for testicular teratoma. The Journal of urology. 1;171(1):161–3.
70. Bodiwala D, Summerton DJ, Terry TR. (2007) Testicular prostheses: development and modern usage. The Annals of The Royal College of Surgeons of England. 89(4):349–53.
71. Warde P, Jewett MA. (1998) Surveillance for stage I testicular seminoma: is it a good option?. Urologic Clinics of North America. 1;25(3):425–33.
72. Warde P, Specht L, Horwich A, et al. (2002) Prognostic factors for relapse in stage I seminoma managed by surveillance: a pooled analysis. Journal of clinical oncology. 5;20(22):4448–52.
73. Cornelison TL, Reed E. (1993) Nephrotoxicity and hydration management for cisplatin, carboplatin, and ormaplatin. Gynecologic oncology. 1;50(2):147–58.
74. Albers P, Albrecht W, Algaba F, et al. (2017) EAU Guidelines on Testicular Cancer. Eur Urol. 71(4):618–629.
75. Khan FA, Kalsi JS. (2018) Testicular Cancer. In: Arya M, Shergill IS, Fernando HS, Kalsi JS, Muneer A, Ahmed HU. Viva Practice for the FRCS (Urol) and Postgraduate Urology Examinations. CRC Press, London.
76. www.cancerresearchuk.org [last accessed 25 May 2020].
77. Maden C, Sherman KJ, Beckmann AM, et al. (1993) History of circumcision, medical conditions, and sexual activity and risk of penile cancer. JNCI: Journal of the National Cancer Institute. 85(1):19–24.
78. Bleeker MC, Heideman DA, Snijders PJ, et al. (2009) Penile cancer: epidemiology, pathogenesis and prevention. World journal of urology. 27(2):141.
79. Pow-Sang MR, Ferreira U, Pow-Sang JM, et al. (2010) Epidemiology and natural history of penile cancer. Urology. 76(2):S2–6.
80. Muneer A, Kayes O, Ahmed HU, et al. (2009) Molecular prognostic factors in penile cancer. World journal of urology. 27(2):161–7.
81. Belville WD, Cohen JA. (1992) Secondary penile malignancies: the spectrum of presentation. Journal of surgical oncology. 51(2):134–7.
82. Minhas S, Manseck A, Watya S, et al. (2010) Penile cancer—prevention and premalignant conditions. Urology. 76(2):S24–35.
83. Hakenburg OW, Comperat E, Minhas S, et al. (2017) EAU Guidelines on Penile Cancer. European Urology. 71(4):1–29.
84. Pandey D, Mahajan V, Kannan RR. (2006) Prognostic factors in node-positive carcinoma of the penis. Journal of surgical oncology. 93(2):133–8.

85. Heyns CF, Fleshner N, Sangar V, et al. (2010) Management of the lymph nodes in penile cancer. Urology. 76(2):S43–57.
86. Lont AP, Kroon BK, Gallee MP, et al. (2007) Pelvic lymph node dissection for penile carcinoma: extent of inguinal lymph node involvement as an indicator for pelvic lymph node involvement and survival. The Journal of urology. 177(3):947–52.
87. Bouchot O, Rigaud J, Maillet F, et al. (2004) Morbidity of inguinal lymphadenectomy for invasive penile carcinoma. European urology. 45(6):761–6.
88. Aleksic I, Rais-Bahrami S, Daugherty M, et al. (2018) Primary urethral carcinoma: A Surveillance, Epidemiology, and End Results data analysis identifying predictors of cancer-specific survival. *Urology annals*, *10*(2), 170.
89. Gakis G, Witjes JA, Bruins M, et al. (2019) EAU Guidelines on Primary Urethral Carcinoma, European Urology. Available at: https://uroweb.org/wp-content/uploads/EAU-Guidelines-on-Primary-Urethral-Carcinoma-2019.pdf [last accessed 24 May 2020].

UROLOGICAL ONCOLOGY 2 MCQS

1. Which of the following regarding abiraterone is false?
   A) It is an oestrogen receptor agonist
   B) It acts as a CYP17 inhibitor
   C) Strong history of cardio-vascular disease is a contraindication
   D) Haematuria is a common side effect
   E) Angina is a common side effect

2. A newly diagnosed patient with prostate cancer has bilateral extra-capsular extension, with involvement of obturator lymph nodes and liver metastasis. What is his correct staging?
   A) T3aN1M1c
   B) T3aN2M1c
   C) T3bN1M1b
   D) T3bN1M1c
   E) T3bN1M1a

3. On which chromosome is PSA encoded?
   A) 13
   B) 15
   C) 17
   D) 19
   E) 21

4. Which of the following is not a criterion as part of the Wilson and Jungner criteria for screening?
   A) Facilities for diagnosis and treatment should be available
   B) The cost of case-finding should be balanced in relation to care cost as a whole
   C) There should be an agreed policy on whom to treat as patients
   D) There should be a recognised mortality rate for the condition
   E) The test should be acceptable to the population

5. Which of the following statements regarding the pathology of prostate cancer is true?
   A) 80–90% are adenocarcinomas
   B) A key feature is absence of staining for basal cell marker p53
   C) Peripheral zone cancers are less commonly associated with seminal vesicle extension
   D) 30–35% of cancers arise in the transitional zone
   E) 5% of cancers arise in the central zone

6. Which of the following statements regarding mpMRI of the prostate is false?

    A) PROMIS study excluded patients with PSA > 15
    B) 1.5T magnet is appropriate for use in this context
    C) Diffusion weighted imaging appears dark in prostate cancer
    D) Water appears dark on T1-imaging
    E) DCE imaging is taken after gadolinium contrast

7. What is the most appropriate type of US probe required to perform TRUS biopsy?

    A) 4.5 MHz
    B) 7.5 MHz
    C) 9 MHz
    D) 11 MHz
    E) 13.5 MHz

8. Regarding radical radiotherapy for prostate cancer, which of the following is not a component of the response to radiation?

    A) Repair
    B) Regeneration
    C) Repopulation
    D) Reassortment
    E) Reoxygenation

9. A patient with prostate cancer has had radical prostatectomy and full staging imaging. Histology shows tumour invading less than half of both lobes, positive lymph nodes were found in both external iliac groups and CT scan did not show any distant metastasis. What is the correct staging for this patient?

    A) T2cN1M0
    B) T2cN2M0
    C) T2bN1M0
    D) T2cN2M1a
    E) T2cN1M1a

10. Which of the following statements regarding brachytherapy for prostate cancer is true?

    A) Large prostate > 30cc is a contra-indication
    B) It is a treatment option in T2c disease
    C) Low-dose brachytherapy uses Ir-192 seeds
    D) High bladder neck is a relative contra-indication
    E) HIFU cannot be used as treatment option if brachytherapy fails

11. The following are all recognised side-effects of goserelin except?
    A) Azotaemia
    B) Alopecia
    C) Arthralgia
    D) Paraesthesia
    E) Prolongation of QT-interval

12. Which of the following is not a parameter of the Briganti nomogram 2018 for predicting lymph node involvement of prosate cancer?
    A) Pre-operative PSA
    B) Maximum diameter of lesion on mpMRI
    C) Percentage of cores with prostate cancer on targeted biopsy
    D) Clinical stage on mpMRI
    E) Gleason grade group at systematic biopsy

13. Below what level of testosterone concentration should be achieved in castration therapy?
    A) < 75mg / mL
    B) < 50mg / mL
    C) < 25ng / dL
    D) < 75ng / dL
    E) < 50ng / dL

14. Regarding the physiology of androgen secretion, which of the following statements is false?
    A) Over-expression of Bcl-2 is associated with hormone refractory prostate cancer
    B) 5-AR type 1 converts testosterone to DHT
    C) The α and ß sub-units of LH are encoded on different chromosomes
    D) Pasqualini syndrome is associated with high LH levels
    E) Leydig cells have a single nucleus

15. Which of the following is not a sex cord stromal tumour?
    A) Leydig cell tumour
    B) Sertoli cell tumour
    C) Adult granulosa cell tumour
    D) Sustentacular cell tumour
    E) Gonadoblastoma

STATION 2: UROLOGICAL ONCOLOGY 2

16. Which of the following regarding Leydig cell tumours is false?
    A) There is no association with undescended testis
    B) 10% are bilateral at presentation
    C) Radiotherapy is ineffective in their treatment
    D) They cause gynaecomastia in adults
    E) Radical orchidectomy is the standard treatment

17. Which of the following regarding half-life of tumour markers for testicular cancer is correct?
    A) 36 hours for ß-HCG and 5 days for α-FP
    B) 5 days for ß-HCG and 36 hours for α-FP
    C) 12 hours for ß-HCG and 3 days for α-FP
    D) 3 days for ß-HCG and 12 hours for α-FP
    E) 24 hours for ß-HCG and 12 hours for α-FP

18. Elevation of LDH is recognised in all of the following conditions except:
    A) Pancreatitis
    B) Haemolytic anaemia
    C) Haemangioblastoma
    D) Acute infectious mononucleosis
    E) Bone fracture

19. What type of US probe transducer is best suited for performing testicular US?
    A) 2–3 kHz
    B) 3–4.5 kHz
    C) 2–3 MHz
    D) 3–4.5 MHz
    E) 7–10 MHz

20. A newly diagnosed patient with testicular cancer has tumour confined to the testis on radical orchidectomy specimen but with evidence of lympho-vascular invasion, CT showing single lymph node metastasis of 3cm in greatest dimension and no distant metastasis. What is the correct staging for this patient?
    A) pT1N1M0
    B) pT2N2M0
    C) pT1N1M0
    D) pT2N2M0
    E) None of the above

21. Which of the following is not an indication to perform a contra-lateral testicular biopsy in a newly diagnosed patient with testicular cancer?
    A) Age < 40 years
    B) Testicular volume < 15mL
    C) History of undescended testis
    D) Johnsen score 1–3
    E) History of sub-fertility

22. Which of the following viruses are not screened prior to referring a patient for sperm banking?
    A) Hepatitis-B antibody
    B) CMV
    C) HIV-1
    D) HIV-2
    E) Hepatitis-C antibody

23. Which of the following statements regarding stage 1 NSGCT is correct?
    A) Induction chemotherapy is x1 cycle BEP
    B) Outside the retroperitoneum, the majority of micro-metastasis at presentation are in the liver
    C) Presence of vascular invasion on histology is associated with relapse risk of ≤ 28%
    D) 20% of recurrences occur after 12 months of treatment
    E) Embryonal component on histology is not an adverse factor

24. A 32 year male with seminoma in intermediate prognosis group has completed course of BEP chemotherapy. Post-treatment CT scan reveals residual 2cm residual volume retro-peritoneal disease. The most appropriate next step is:
    A) Continue surveillance
    B) Refer for PET scan
    C) Refer for RPLND
    D) Refer for biopsy of residual mass
    E) Give further chemotherapy

25. Regarding stage 1 seminoma, which of the following is false:
    A) Tumour size > 5cm is a risk factor
    B) Rete testis involvement is a risk factor
    C) Rete testis involvement alone has 16% risk of relapse
    D) No risk factors present has 12% risk of relapse
    E) None of the above

26. Regarding stage 1 seminoma, which of the following is true:
    A) For tumours confined to the testis, relapses after 5 years are very rare
    B) Adjuvant radiotherapy causes long term bowel irritation in 20%
    C) Adjuvant radiotherapy is prescribed as 20Gy over 10 fractions
    D) Single dose cisplatin is advised if risk factors present
    E) None of the above

27. Which of the following is false regarding ITGCN?
    A) Histology most commonly shows germ cells with enlarged hyperchromatic nuclei
    B) It is present up to 15% of the contra-lateral testes if all risk factors are present
    C) Cells are typically arranged along the basement membrane of the tubule
    D) Yolk sac tumours do not arise from ITGCN
    E) Spermatocytic seminoma do not arise from ITGCN

28. Which of the following is not a risk factor for SCCa of the penis?
    A) HPV 18
    B) HIV
    C) UVA light
    D) UVB light
    E) Lymphoma

29. A 72 year male with type-2 diabetes and HIV presents to you with a painful blue papule on the penis. The most likely diagnosis is:
    A) Kaposi's sarcoma
    B) Primary syphilis
    C) Buschke-Lowenstein tumour
    D) Bowenoid papulosis
    E) Verrucous carcinoma

30. A newly diagnosed patient with penile cancer has histology showing sub-epithelial connective tissue invasion and Grade 2 SCCa, with CT showing metastasis in 5 unilateral inguinal nodes and lung metastasis. What is the correct staging?
    A) T1aN1M1a
    B) T1aN2M1a
    C) T1bN1M1a
    D) T1bN2M1a
    E) None of the above

31. A newly diagnosed patient with penile cancer has histology showing tumour invading both corpus spongiosum, 3 positive bilateral inguinal lymph nodes on radical lymphadenectomy specimen and no distant metastasis on CT. What is the correct staging?
    A) T1bN2M0
    B) T2pN3M0
    C) T2pN2M0
    D) T3pN2M0
    E) T3pN3M0

32. Which of the following imiquimod is false?
    A) A standard course is 4–6 weeks
    B) Asthenia is a common side effect
    C) Patient should avoid having sexual intercourse during treatment
    D) Circumcision should be performed prior to offering treatment
    E) None of the above

33. Which of the following statements regarding the boundaries of the pelvic lymphadenectomy operation is false?
    A) Inferior margin is Cloquet's node
    B) Lateral margin is genito-femoral nerve
    C) Medial margin is bladder wall
    D) Superior margin is obturator nerve
    E) Proximal margin is iliac bifurcation

34. A newly diagnosed patient with penile cancer has histology showing invasion of sub-epithelial connective tissue with lympho-vascular invasion and Grade 1 SCC, there are no palpable lymph nodes and no enlarged nodes or distant metastasis on staging CT. What is the most appropriate next step?
    A) Offer surveillance
    B) Refer for US and FNA
    C) Refer for DSNB
    D) Refer for modified inguinal lymphadenectomy
    E) Refer for radical inguinal lymphadenectomy

35. Which factor in penile cancer histology does not increase the risk of lymph node involvement?
    A) Sarcomatoid variant
    B) Helical growth pattern
    C) Urethral invasion
    D) Lympho-vascular invasion
    E) ≥ Grade 3 disease

STATION 3
PAEDIATRIC UROLOGY

ANTENATAL HYDRONEPHROSIS

VESICO-URETERIC REFLUX

POSTERIOR URETHRAL VALVES

PELVIURETERIC JUNCTION OBSTRUCTION

ECTOPIC URETER, URETEROCOELE AND RENAL DYSPLASIA

PHIMOSIS AND CIRCUMCISION

UNDESCENDED TESTIS

HYPOSPADIAS

PAEDIATRIC HYDROCOELE

DAY-TIME LOWER URINARY TRACT CONDITIONS

MONOSYMPTOMATIC NOCTURNAL ENURESIS

URINARY TRACT INFECTIONS IN CHILDREN

DISORDERS OF SEXUAL DEVELOPMENT

MISCELLANEOUS PAEDIATRIC UROLOGY

CONTENTS

ANTENATAL HYDRONEPHROSIS   175
  EPIDEMIOLOGY   175
  AETIOLOGY   175
  ANTENATAL MANAGEMENT   175
  POSTNATAL MANAGEMENT   176

VESICO-URETERIC REFLUX   **178**
  EPIDEMIOLOGY   178
  PATHOGENESIS   178
  CLASSIFICATION   179
  GRADING   179
  PRESENTATION   180
  DIAGNOSTIC EVALUATION   181
    IMAGING   181
  MANAGEMENT   182
    CONSERVATIVE THERAPY   182
    SURGICAL TREATMENT   183

POSTERIOR URETHRAL VALVES   **185**
  EPIDEMIOLOGY   185
  PATHOLOGY   185
  CLASSIFICATION   185
  PRESENTATION   185
  MANAGEMENT   186
    ANTENATAL MANAGEMENT   186
    POST-NATAL MANAGEMENT   186
  FOLLOW-UP   187

PELVIURETERIC JUNCTION OBSTRUCTION   **188**
  EPIDEMIOLOGY   188
  AETIOLOGY   188
  PRESENTATION   188
  INVESTIGATION   188
  MANAGEMENT   188
  MEGA-URETER   189

CLASSIFICATION	189
EPIDEMIOLOGY	189
AETIOLOGY	190
INVESTIGATION	190
MANAGEMENT	190
ECTOPIC URETER, URETEROCOELE AND RENAL DYSPLASIA	**191**
ECTOPIC URETER	191
EPIDEMIOLOGY	191
CLASSIFICATION	191
PRESENTATION	191
INVESTIGATION	191
MANAGEMENT	192
URETEROCOELE	192
EPIDEMIOLOGY	192
CLASSIFICATION	192
PRESENTATION	192
INVESTIGATION	193
MANAGEMENT	193
RENAL DYSPLASIA	193
HORSESHOE KIDNEY	193
ECTOPIC KIDNEY	194
RENAL AGENESIS	194
DUPLEX KIDNEY	194
PHIMOSIS AND CIRCUMCISION	**195**
EPIDEMIOLOGY	195
PHYSIOLOGICAL PHIMOSIS	195
BALANITIS XEROTICA OBLITERANS	195
CIRCUMCISION	196
PREPUTIOPLASTY	196
BURIED PENIS MEGAPREPUCE	196
UNDESCENDED TESTIS	**198**
EPIDEMIOLOGY	198
AETIOLOGY	198

RISK FACTORS	198
CLASSIFICATION	198
DIAGNOSTIC EVALUATION	200
MANAGEMENT	200
INGUINAL ORCHIDOPEXY	201
NON-PALPABLE TESTIS MANAGEMENT	202
MANAGEMENT OF OLDER PATIENTS	204
HYPOSPADIAS	**205**
EPIDEMIOLOGY	205
CLASSIFICATION	205
AETIOLOGY	205
ASSOCIATED ABNORMALITIES	206
DIAGNOSTIC EVALUATION	206
MANAGEMENT	206
CORRECTION OF CURVATURE	207
DEALING WITH HOODED FORESKIN	207
RE-SITING URETHRAL MEATUS	208
COMPLICATIONS	208
PAEDIATRIC HYDROCOELE	**209**
PRIMARY HYDROCOELE	209
SECONDARY HYDROCOELE	209
DIAGNOSTIC EVALUATION	210
MANAGEMENT	210
DAY-TIME LOWER URINARY TRACT CONDITIONS	**211**
CLASSIFICATION	211
DIAGNOSTIC EVALUATION	213
HISTORY	213
EXAMINATION	214
IMAGING	214
MANAGEMENT	214
MONOSYMPTOMATIC NOCTURNAL ENURESIS	**216**
EPIDEMIOLOGY	216
PATHOPHYSIOLOGY	216

DIAGNOSTIC EVALUATION	216
HISTORY	217
EXAMINATION	217
MANAGEMENT	217
URINARY TRACT INFECTIONS IN CHILDREN	**219**
EPIDEMIOLOGY	219
CLASSIFICATION	219
DIAGNOSTIC EVALUATION	220
IMAGING	221
MANAGEMENT	222
DISORDERS OF SEXUAL DEVELOPMENT	**223**
EVALUATION	223
SEX CHROMOSOME DSD	224
KLINEFELTER'S SYNDROME (47 XXY)	224
TURNER'S SYNDROME	225
MIXED GONADAL DYSGENESIS	225
VIRILISATION OF 46XX FEMALE (46 XX DSD)	226
CONGENITAL ADRENAL HYPERPLASIA	226
INADEQUATE VIRILISATION OF 46 XY MALE (46 XY DSD)	226
COMPLETE ANDROGEN INSENSITIVITY SYNDROME	226
5α – REDUCTASE DEFICIENCY	227
MISCELLANEOUS PAEDIATRIC UROLOGY	**228**
EMBRYOLOGY OF KIDNEY	228
PAEDIATRIC FLUIDS	228
WILMS' TUMOUR	228
EPIDEMIOLOGY	228
PATHOLOGY	229
DIAGNOSTIC EVALUATION	229
MANAGEMENT	229
RHABDOMYOSARCOMA	230
NEUROBLASTOMA	230
PRUNE BELLY SYNDROME	230
PAEDIATRIC UROLOGY MCQS	**231**
REFERENCES	**237**

ANTENATAL HYDRONEPHROSIS

EPIDEMIOLOGY

Use of US during pregnancy has yielded higher detection rate for antenatal hydronephrosis.

Incidence is 0.6% on second trimester (20 weeks gestation). [1]

65% of cases will resolve without treatment and < 5% require surgical intervention.

Recall that minimum standard antenatal scans performed in the NHS are at 12 and 20 weeks gestation.

AETIOLOGY

The following are all potential causes of antenatal hydronephrosis:

PUJO (most common cause), VUR, megaureter, PUV, ureterocoele, renal cysts, MCDK, physiological hydronephrosis. [2]

These conditions will be covered individually in their appropriate stations.

ANTENATAL MANAGEMENT

Kidneys can be visualised clearly at 20 weeks gestation (NHS anomaly scan), when almost all the amniotic fluid is urine.

The most sensitive time for foetal urinary tract assessment is at 28 weeks gestation (i.e. if a repeat US is planned following detection of abnormality).

The following information must be obtained from antenatal US:
- degree of hydronephrosis (APD renal pelvis > 5mm)
- cortical thinning and echogenicity of renal parenchyma
- ureteric assessment for dilatation
- bladder assessment for thickness, emptying or not seen (bladder exstrophy)
- visible penis to determine male gender
- amniotic fluid volume (oligo- or an- hydramnios is a marker of poor outcome)

US should be repeated later in 3rd trimester of pregnancy to review progression of hydronephrosis.

Counselling, important for expectations particularly for severe cases with massive progressive bilateral dilatation, oligo- / an- hydramnios and pulmonary hypoplasia.

Delivery, in high-risk cases should be planned in appropriate tertiary centre with neonatal ITU.

Intra-uterine intervention is rarely indicated.

POSTNATAL MANAGEMENT

Post-natal investigation and management of antenatal hydronephrosis will depend on underlying diagnosis and severity, and are described in appropriate stations of the various pathologies.

Clinical assessment including BP measurement.

Blood tests to include kidney function and arterial blood gas sampling where appropriate.

Consider starting antibiotic prophylaxis (trimethoprim 2mg / kg OD).

Post-Natal US

Transitory neonatal dehydration lasts 48 hours after birth, therefore post-natal US should be deferred following this period of neonatal oliguria (repeat 1–2 weeks post-partum).

Immediate post-natal US is however warranted in severe cases (oligo-hydramnios, solitary kidney, bilateral obstruction).

Post-Natal Micturating Cysto-Urethrogram

MCUG can be deferred until the child is older in non-urgent clinical scenarios (e.g. VUR).

In urgent cases the MCUG should be performed as soon as possible after birth (e.g. suspected PUV in the context of bilateral hydro-uretero nephrosis and thick-walled bladder).

DMSA / MAG-3 Renogram

Usually deferred until child is > 6 weeks of age

Figure 1 – Algorithm for antenatal hydronephrosis]

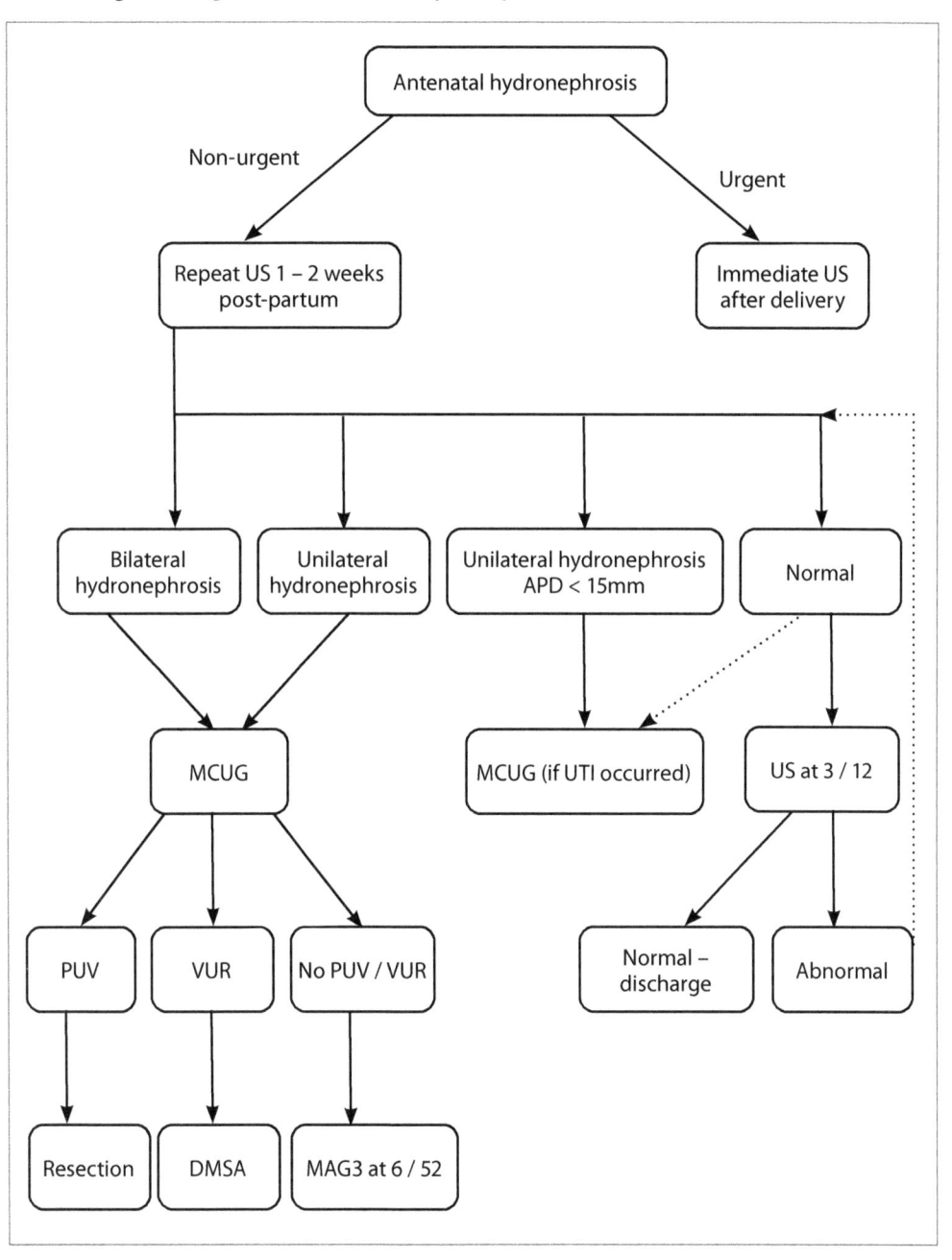

VESICO-URETERIC REFLUX

VUR is an anatomical and / or functional disorder resulting from abnormal retrograde flow of urine from the bladder into the upper urinary tract.

EPIDEMIOLOGY

Overall incidence in children is 1%.

Incidence greater in white vs. black African females.

Offspring of affected parent have 40% incidence of VUR, siblings of affected child have 30% risk of reflux – however screening remains controversial (e.g. US as screening tool). [3]

Sibling screening is challenging due to lack of non-invasive tests (MCUG requires catheterisation).

Female to male ratio is 5 : 1.

VUR in males tends to be diagnosed at younger age (0–2 years) and be of a higher grade but has a greater chance of spontaneous resolution. [4]

VUR in females tends to be diagnosed later (2–7 years) but be of lower grade severity.

Incidence of VUR in children with UTIs is 30% and in antenatal hydronephrosis is 15%.

Reflux nephropathy is one of the commonest causes of hypertension in children.

PATHOGENESIS

Anti-reflux mechanisms include the oblique entry of ureter through bladder wall (1–2 cm) and muscular attachments which prevent reflux during bladder filling and voiding.

VUR arises from deficiency of valvular mechanism of longitudinal muscle of intra-vesical ureter.

The normal ratio of intra-mural ureteric length to ureteric diameter is 5 : 1.

Paquin's law, where reflux occurs due to short intra-mural length (ratio < 5 : 1).

CLASSIFICATION

Primary

Results from congenital abnormality of the VUJ (e.g. Paquin's law).

In duplication, the Weigert-Meyer rule states the lower moiety ureter enters the bladder proximally and laterally, resulting in shorter intra-mural length and thus higher risk of reflux.

Genetically recognised cause with autosomal dominant inheritance.

Secondary

Results from urinary tract dysfunction associated with elevated intra-vesical pressures (VUR tends to resolve once bladder pressures brought down to normal).

Reflux of sterile urine at physiological voiding pressures does not cause renal scarring.

The most common anatomic bladder obstruction causing VUR in boys are PUV, and VUR is present in a majority of patients with this condition.

In females the most common anatomical cause is ureterocoele.

Neuropathic bladders with intra-vesical pressures > 40cm H_2O have strong association with VUR.

Other causes include PUV, DSD, urethral stenosis.

Treatment for secondary reflux is to target the underlying cause.

GRADING

Grading is based on the extent of retrograde filling and dilatation of the ureter, renal pelvis and calyces on MCUG (accurately grading reflux in impossible with co-existent ipsilateral obstruction).

Table 1 – Grading system for VUR on MCUG according to International Reflux Study Committee [2]

VUR Grade	Characteristics	Rate of spontaneous resolution (%)	Distribution of Grades (%)
1	Reflux does not reach renal pelvis with varying degrees of ureteral dilatation	90	7
2	Reflux reaches renal pelvis, no dilatation of collecting system, normal fornices	80	53
3	Mild/moderate ureteric dilatation +/- tortuosity, moderate dilatation of collecting system, normal or minimally deformed fornices	50	32
4	Moderate ureteric dilatation +/- tortuosity, moderate dilatation of collecting system, blunt fornices, papillae impressions still visible	20	6
5	Gross ureteric dilatation and tortuosity, marked dilatation of collecting system, papillary impressions not visible, intra-parenchymal reflux	< 10	2

PRESENTATION

VUR may present with a wide range of severity, however most do not feature renal scarring and do not require any surgical intervention.

Asymptomatic bacteriuria is not associated with renal scarring.

VUR may present acutely with UTI, failure to thrive or even chronic vomiting and diarrhoea.

Pyelonephritis in children may result in renal scarring (however rarely resulting in renal impairment) which does carry a long-term risk of hypertension (10% if unilateral, 20% if bilateral).

Greatest risk of renal scarring is < 4 years of age (as intra-mural ureter elongates with growth), scarring occurs maximally after 1st episode of pyelonephritis.

Having VUR that is symptomatic (i.e. UTI) increases risk of scarring. [5]

Acute pyelonephritis in children has 20% risk of recurrence within 12 months.

VUR may also present with LUT dysfunction (LUTD), including urge +/- incontinence, frequency, prolonged voiding or even bowel dysfunction.

VUR is the most common cause of severe hypertension in children and young adults.

DIAGNOSTIC EVALUATION

History from the parent and / or child should enquire regarding:
- overall health and development of child
- presence of LUTD, UTI
- parental and sibling history of VUR

Examination of the child should cover:
- general examination of height, weight (growth chart)
- urological assessment for palpable bladder or kidneys, external genitalia
- BP, urinalysis and culture

Blood tests may include UE if bilateral renal cortical abnormalities.

IMAGING

MCUG is gold-standard investigation to diagnose VUR, assess grade and reversible causes. [6]
- patient is catheterised and iodine-based contrast injected into bladder
- x-rays are taken and catheter is then removed
- patient voids and x-rays taken again

DMSA renogram is useful in assessment of VUR for:
- detecting renal cortical scarring (photo-deficient lesions)
- baseline DMSA at diagnosis used for comparison with successive scans for follow-up
- split kidney function
- diagnostic tool during suspected acute pyelonephritis (dimercaptosuccinic acid uptake is poor in areas of inflammation and will appear as cold-spots)

VUDS not routinely used unless underlying secondary reflux is suspected e.g. spina bifida, PUV.

US can be used as a 1st standard evaluation tool for antenatal hydronephrosis, repeated > 7 days after birth.

US can reliably assess kidney size, collecting system dilatation and parenchymal thickness.

US is not sensitive for VUR; absent hydronephrosis does not exclude VUR however 2 normal sequential US make significant VUR unlikely.

The presence of cortical scarring on US warrants further assessment with MCUG.

MANAGEMENT

The main management goal is preservation of kidney function by minimising pyelonephritis risk.

Risk factors for each patient (age, sex, grade of reflux, associated LUTD, abnormal anatomy and kidney appearance) should be evaluated to identify those at highest risk of scarring.

The majority of primary VUR grades I–II will resolve spontaneously (80%)

Overall 50% resolution seen in grades III–V as child's growth elongates the intra-mural segment of ureter, within 4–5 years follow up.

CONSERVATIVE THERAPY

General advice, includes good fluid intake, treatment of any constipation, regular voiding.

Education includes parental awareness of urgency to treat UTI or febrile presentations.

Prophylactic antibiotics (CAP), not required for low-grade reflux however a safe approach would be to consider CAP in most cases, mandatory in VUR with LUTD.

CAP should be continued until child is toilet trained.

Whilst on conservative treatment, growth, BP and urinalysis should be monitored + annual US.

RIVUR Trial [7]

Randomised, placebo-controlled trial published in NEJM (2014) regarding anti-microbial prophylaxis for children with vesico-ureteric reflux

600+ children with VUR randomised to receive antibiotic prophylaxis vs. placebo

Found reduced risk of recurrent UTI by 50% but not renal scarring and its consequences (hypertension, ESRF) and increased anti-microbial resistance.

Swedish Reflux Study [8]

Evaluated > 200 children with grade 3–4 VUR randomised equally to:

    prophylactic antibiotics vs. endoscopic injection vs. surveillance

MCUG and DMSA performed before randomisation and after 2 years.

Findings: Girls – prophylactic antibiotics reduced scarring and UTI, injections reduced UTI

    Boys – no benefit from any active treatment

SURGICAL TREATMENT

The indications for surgical treatment for VUR include:
- failure of conservative therapy (breakthrough UTI, non-compliance, new renal scarring)
- persistent high-grade (IV or V) VUR

There is no consensus regarding optimum timing of surgical correction.

Circumcision may be beneficial in males with VUR and anatomical abnormalities.

Endoscopic Options

Day-case cystoscopy and injection of bulking agent Deflux around the ureteric orifice with success rates of 80% (can be repeated). [9]

Sub-ureteric Teflon injection (STING) fallen out of favour due to Teflon migration to distant organs.

Open Surgery Options

There are various options involving re-implantation of the ureter: [9]

- *intra-vesical*, by opening the bladder, mobilising the ureter and advancing it across the trigone (Cohen's repair) or implanting it higher and more medially (Leadbetter-Politano repair) always respecting the 5 : 1 Paquin's rule
- *extra-vesical*, by suturing the distal ureter onto the bladder and constructing a tunnel of detrusor muscle around it (Lich-Gregoir procedure)

POSTERIOR URETHRAL VALVES

EPIDEMIOLOGY

PUV are one of the few life-threatening congenital abnormalities of the urinary tract found during neonatal period.

Alternative term is Congenital Obstructive Posterior Urethral Membrane (COPUM).

Incidence of 1 in 5000 males [10]

50% will have day- and night-time incontinence at age 5 years.

By age 20 years, 50% will have chronic kidney disease and 1 / 3 ESRF. [11]

PATHOLOGY

PUV arise through abnormal Wolffian duct insertion in urogenital sinus during foetal development (it does not occur in females).

Outflow obstruction leads to abnormalities in bladder wall components (increased collagen content, aberrations in nerve supply and renal dysplasia).

CLASSIFICATION

PUV were originally described by H.H.Young into three categories: [12]

- *Type 1*, bicuspid valves from verumontanum through to membranous urethra, fusing with anterior wall of urethra
- *Type 2*, is a fold and non-obstructive and therefore not associated with PUV
- *Type 3*, sheet membrane attached to entire urethral circumference with a central aperture (iris-shaped), this will be converted to type-1 when a catheter is passed

PRESENTATION

The majority are diagnosed antenatally – 60% identified on US at 20 weeks gestation (accounting for 1% of all antenatal hydronephrosis cases).

Antenatal US findings include:
- bilateral hydro-uretero nephrosis
- thick-walled bladder

- dilated posterior urethra (keyhole sign)
- renal dysplasia
- oligo-hydramnios

Newborns / infants may present with urinary sepsis, palpable bladder, signs of renal failure and respiratory distress secondary to pulmonary hypoplasia (most common cause of early mortality).

Potter's facies, (due to oligo-hydramnios) include flattened nose, epicanthal folds, low-set ears.

Older children may present as milder cases with recurrent UTI, weak stream, incontinence, failure to thrive and renal failure.

Pop-off valve syndrome, is a self-defence mechanism to reduce high urinary tract pressure by leaking urine from a bladder or renal pelvis rupture (urinary ascites), diverticula or reflux into kidney (thus protecting contra-lateral kidney) (not known to preserve overall long term renal function). [13]

This will be noted as extravasation on the MCUG.

MANAGEMENT

ANTENATAL MANAGEMENT

The placement of vesico-amniotic shunt does not make a difference to long term outcome in PUV.

LASER ablation of foetal valves is only to be considered experimental.

Consider repeat antenatal US to review progression in 3rd trimester – if bilateral / severe, plan for delivery in tertiary centre with neonatal ITU / nephrology.

POST-NATAL MANAGEMENT

Resuscitate in a systematic fashion following Airway to Exposure protocol, with paediatric support at hand and access to neonatal ITU.

The following aspects of management must be addressed:

- *catheter insertion*, using 6F feeding tube (although the risk of this is that it may fall out) or a SPC, (risk of urethral catheter is balloon inflation may occlude ureteric orifices)
- *treat diuresis*, by replacing fluids, monitoring urine output and UEs, liaise with nephrology

- *prophylactic antibiotics*, e.g. trimethoprim 2mg / kg daily
- urgent imaging to include repeat US and proceeding to MCUG

Once emergency management is in place, proceed to establish a diagnosis.

The investigation of choice is the MCUG. [2]

On the MCUG in PUV a secondary reflux is observed in > 50% (associated with renal dysplasia) and it is important to check catheter is in bladder and not posterior urethra. [14]

MCUG may show dilated ureter, trabeculated bladder, narrowed junction between dilated posterior urethra and narrower anterior urethra (site of PUV).

Valve Ablation

Definitive treatment is cystoscopy and ablation / resection of valves under general anaesthesia.

Main complication is urethral stricture (i.e. limit electrocoagulation and use cold knife). [15]

If the urethra is too small to allow cystoscope, a temporary vesicostomy is performed (unless SPC already in situ which can be left up to 12 weeks).

FOLLOW-UP

Following valve resection, a follow-up cystoscopy or MCUG should be repeated at 3 months, to assess for any residual valve tissue.

DMSA should be performed to assess split kidney function. [2]

VUDS should be considered to assess any voiding dysfunction in childhood.

Despite early intervention, bladder function is abnormal in 70% of boys in the long term (consider stating in the FRCS (Urol) viva that you would never discharge a boy with PUV).

Long-term follow-up is warranted due to implications of PUV – renal function monitoring, assessments of LUTS conditions, recurrent UTI and overall development.

Poor prognosis associated with oligo-hydramnios, high levels B2 micro globulin in foetal urine (antenatally) and low GFR, daytime incontinence, urodynamic detrusor failure (postnatally).

PELVIURETERIC JUNCTION OBSTRUCTION

EPIDEMIOLOGY

Childhood incidence is 1 in a 1000.

Boys : Girls ratio is 2 : 1, left : right ratio is 2 : 1, bilateral in 10%. [16]

AETIOLOGY

In most children the PUJO is congenital.

Extrinsic, due to compression of PUJ by aberrant crossing vessels.

Intrinsic, due to abnormal insertion of ureter into renal pelvis, ureteric folds or PUJ muscle which is hypo-plastic or aperistaltic.

PRESENTATION

Most commonly diagnosed via antenatal US with unilateral hydronephrosis (PUJO is most common cause of hydronephrosis without ureteric dilatation).

UTI, haematuria, loin pain or palpable mass

Deitl's crisis, pain exacerbated by drinking large fluid volumes where subsequent diuresis exacerbates stretching of the upper tract. [17]

INVESTIGATION

US allows assessment of degree of hydronephrosis, calyceal dilatation and cortical thinning.

US should be repeated urgently after birth (if severe bilateral hydronephrosis), for non-urgent cases defer > 7 days to allow physiological diuresis which may resolve hydronephrosis.

If US excludes ureteric dilatation then there is no need for MCUG.

MAG-3 renogram is performed at 6–12 weeks to clinch the diagnosis.

MANAGEMENT

Conservative treatment with antibiotic prophylaxis cover is warranted until diagnosis made.

The mainstay of treatment is pyeloplasty surgery – which can be achieved laparoscopically (Anderson-Hynes dismembered) or open, with equal long-term outcomes.

Minimally invasive improves cosmesis, in-patient hospital stay and complication rates.

The following are indications for surgery: [2]

- symptomatic children
- reduced function of kidney (< 40% is significant)
- deteriorating affected kidney function (decrease in > 10% differential function or increasing hydronephrosis on US
- hydronephrosis > 50 mm of renal AP pelvic diameter

If the kidney is non-functional then a nephrectomy is advised.

Most children with an APD renal pelvis > 40mm will require surgery, however only 1–3% of those with APD < 20mm require this (20% of those 20–30mm). [9]

MEGA-URETER

Mega-ureter is the term to describe a dilated ureter (> 7mm) which may be a primary condition or secondary to any other condition with may dilate the ureter.

Secondary mega-ureter may be due to stone passage, tumour or BOO (if bilateral).

CLASSIFICATION

Mega-ureter can be divided into 4 groups:

- obstructed
- non-refluxing, non-obstructed
- refluxing
- refluxing and obstructed

EPIDEMIOLOGY

Affects 1 in 200 children, boys more frequently than girls, left more than right.

4% of cases of antenatally detected hydronephrosis.

The most common presenting symptom is UTI.

AETIOLOGY

Refluxing mega-ureter is due to VUR (discussed in "Vesico-ureteric reflux" section).

Obstructive mega-ureter is associated with a stenotic or aperistaltic segment of distal ureter.

INVESTIGATION

US should be repeated > 7 days after birth to reassess persistence of ureteric dilatation.

MCUG can help distinguish between obstructive and refluxing cause.

MAG-3 may be performed 6–12 weeks after delivery (ipsilateral PUJO is found in 13% of cases) and can help distinguish obstructed vs. non-obstructed.

MANAGEMENT

Principles are similar as per PUJO surgical strategy.

Conservative treatment is warranted with antibiotic prophylaxis, providing child is symptom-free, split function > 40% and no deterioration in sonographic / renogram tests.

Surgery < 12 months of age is usually limited to stent insertion.

Definitive surgery includes ureteric re-implantation +/- excision of stenotic segment of ureter.

ECTOPIC URETER, URETEROCOELE AND RENAL DYSPLASIA

ECTOPIC URETER

EPIDEMIOLOGY

Ectopic ureter is caused by the ureteric bud which arises from an abnormally high or low position on the mesonephric duct during embryological development.

80% are associated with a duplicated collection system.

Incidence is 1 : 2000 and is 3x more common in females.

Most ectopic ureters in females are associated with a duplex kidney.

Most common site for ectopic ureter drainage in boys is the posterior urethra.

CLASSIFICATION

Two ureters may join to form a single ureter, or they may both pass down individually into the bladder (complete duplication).

Weigert-Meyer rule, in the case of complete duplication the upper renal moiety always opens onto the bladder below and medial to the lower moiety ureter.

i.e. the upper moiety obstructs, the lower moiety refluxes.

PRESENTATION

Antenatally – with US detected hydronephrosis

Postnatally – with acute or recurrent UTI, dribbling of urine, epididymitis (in pre-adolescent boys)

Females – if the ureteric opening is below the urethral sphincter, will present with persistent incontinence (this does not occur in males).

INVESTIGATION

US for initial assessment, MCUG evaluates for reflux.

DMSA assess split function and differential function between upper and lower pole moieties of a duplex kidney to help plan surgery.

MANAGEMENT

Conservative with prophylactic antibiotic cover is an option in the well-child.

An ectopic ureter associated with dilated poorly functioning upper moiety of kidney is an indication for hemi-nephrectomy.

URETEROCOELE

EPIDEMIOLOGY

A ureterocoele is a cystic dilatation of the distal intra-vesical ureter as it drains into the bladder.

Female to male ratio is 4 : 1.

80% associated with upper pole ureter in duplicated systems, 20% in single systems, 10% are bilateral.

CLASSIFICATION

Intravesical / Orthotopic (20%): [2]

Ureterocoele completely confined within the bladder, more common in males and single system

- stenotic, small stenotic ureteric orifice associated with obstruction
- non-obstructed, large ureteric orifice

Extravesical / Ectopic (80%): [2]

Ureterocoele extends to bladder neck or urethra, more common in females and duplex systems

- sphincteric (extends into bladder neck and urethra)
- sphinctero-stenotic (ureteric orifice stenosed)
- caeco-ureterocoele
- blind ectopic

PRESENTATION

Antenatally – with US detected hydronephrosis, postnatally – with UTI, pain, vaginal mass in girls (if prolapsing ureterocoele)

Ureterocoeles usually cause obstruction of the upper pole.

INVESTIGATION

US shows a thin-walled cyst in the bladder.

MCUG identifies ureterocoele location, size, associated VUR.

DMSA for renal moiety function and cortical abnormalities in the presence of VUR.

MANAGEMENT

Commence treatment with antibiotic prophylaxis at birth.

The choice of treatment modality depends on the following criteria:
- clinical status of patient
- age of child
- presence of reflux or obstruction
- function of upper pole
- intra-vesical vs. ectopic ureterocoele

Management is controversial with a choice between conservative, endoscopic decompression, ureteral reimplantation, partial nephroureterectomy or complete reconstruction.

Early treatment – antibiotics, immediate endoscopic incision of ureterocoele if septic or if featuring bladder neck obstruction.

Re-evaluation – appropriate if child is asymptomatic, no severe hydro-uretero-nephrosis and no evidence of bladder outlet obstruction.

Surgery may vary from upper pole nephrectomy to complete ipsilateral LUT reconstruction.

RENAL DYSPLASIA

HORSESHOE KIDNEY

Horseshoe kidney is the most common example of renal fusion – prevalence 1 in 400. [18]

The kidneys lie vertically rather than obliquely and are joined by an isthmus (located anterior to L3 – L4) which in 95% of cases joins the lower poles.

Ascent of the kidney is obstructed by the inferior mesenteric artery; hence it lies lower in the abdomen.

Normal rotation is prevented, therefore renal pelvis lies anteriorly and ureters pass anteriorly over the kidneys and isthmus.

Most patients are asymptomatic with a normal renal function.

Horseshoe kidney in presence of coarctation of aorta may suggest Turner's syndrome. [19]

ECTOPIC KIDNEY

Kidneys fail to achieve normal position, and can be thoracic, abdominal, pelvic or lumbar.

The affected kidney is usually smaller.

Left is more common than right, bilateral in < 10%.

Pelvic location is most common (60%) and most frequent cause of hydronephrosis in this scenario is due to PUJO – as a result of incomplete rotation of kidney.

Pelvic kidneys lie opposite the sacrum and below the bifurcation of the aorta.

RENAL AGENESIS

Unilateral renal agenesis is the absence of one kidney due to embryological abnormality or absence of the ureteric bud (failed induction of nephrogenesis).

Incidence of unilateral renal agenesis is 1 : 1000 (left more than right, males more than females).

Many patients are asymptomatic.

Associated with absent ipsilateral ureter, uterine abnormalities (unicornuate, where one side failed to develop; didelphys, double uterus), absence of vas deferens.

Bilateral renal agenesis affects males in 75% of cases and is incompatible with life.

DUPLEX KIDNEY

Duplex kidneys arise from two separate ureteric buds which induce separate segments of the metanephric blastema.

PUJO and VUR most commonly occur in the duplex lower pole.

Ectopic ureter is almost always associated with the duplex upper pole.

PHIMOSIS AND CIRCUMCISION

EPIDEMIOLOGY

By 12 months of age, foreskin retraction behind glanular sulcus is achieved in 50%, therefore in those where this is not possible it is termed "physiological".

Phimosis is present in 8% of 6 year olds and 1% of 16 year olds (i.e. most cases will resolve). [20]

PHYSIOLOGICAL PHIMOSIS

Physiological phimosis can be also termed primary phimosis.

This arises due to adhesions between the glans epithelium with the inner epithelium lining layer.

Physiological phimosis should resolve naturally by processes which separate these layers of skin:

- spontaneous erections
- penile growth
- epithelial desquamation

Non-surgical treatment includes 6 weeks of twice daily betamethasone valerate 0.1% (betnovate) applied topically as steroid (no long-term demonstrable risks or side-effects) success rate reported 90% and therefore indicated as 1st line treatment. [2]

BALANITIS XEROTICA OBLITERANS

BXO is also known as lichen sclerosus and can affect any skin part but has a predilection for genitalia.

Cardinal signs on histology include loss of rete pegs, hyper-keratosis and thinned epithelium.

BXO is not contagious. The pathophysiology remains unknown however auto-immune mechanism has been suggested as well as a sequalae of chronic infections.

Can affect glans, foreskin, external urethral meatus and urethra.

Examination when retracting the foreskin will reveal a white thickened ring of tissue, rather than the pink inner mucosa of foreskin which should appear as a carnation flower.

BXO is not corrected by topical steroids or preputioplasty but requires a circumcision.

CIRCUMCISION

The indications for circumcision include:
- treatment of BXO [2]
- recurrent symptomatic balanoposthitis

Circumcision can also contribute in the management plan of children with vesico-ureteric reflux (NNT to prevent 1 UTI is 4) and recurrent UTI (NNT to prevent 1 UTI is 11). [9]

Routine neonatal circumcision is not recommended to prevent penile carcinoma. [21]

Circumcision contraindicated in:
- presence of hypospadias (foreskin required for reconstruction)
- active balanitis
- buried penis mega-prepuce
- uncorrected coagulopathy

Risks include infection requiring antibiotics (2%), bleeding and return to theatre (1%), cosmetic dissatisfaction, meatal stenosis, urethrocutaneous fistula.

PREPUTIOPLASTY

Longitudinal preputial incision sutured transversely in the aim of widening the preputial opening.

Not a treatment for BXO.

Requires child co-operation to regularly retract foreskin after surgery and maintain hygiene.

BURIED PENIS MEGAPREPUCE

Also known as congenital mega-prepuce.

Patients will present with buried penis, whereby outer preputial skin appears to meet directly with abdominal wall skin dorsally and scrotum ventrally. [22]

It is not a true phimosis.

Urine collects in foreskin and has to be milked out.

Surgical correction involves removing the inner preputial skin and using the outer preputial skin to substitute penile shaft.

Mega-meatus is congenital appearance of a large meatus; patient can be discharged.

UNDESCENDED TESTIS

EPIDEMIOLOGY

Cryptorchidism or UDT is one of the most common congenital malformations of male neonates.

4% of full-term births – many will spontaneously descend, therefore incidence at 1 year is 1% (most will have descended by 3 months of age due to neonatal LH surge).

i.e. if not descended by 3 months, it is unlikely to occur spontaneously

Significantly more common in pre-term infants (40%).

Occurs bilaterally in 30% of cases – undertake thorough examination to assess for DSD.

AETIOLOGY

Until 6 weeks gestation the gonads remain undifferentiated (until SRY gene influence occurs).

SRY is the master gene responsible for male sexual differentiation. [9]

1st Phase (7–8 weeks) – testicular descent from genital ridge to internal inguinal ring, occurs under influence of MIS.

2nd Phase (25–30 weeks) – testicular descent through inguinal canal into scrotum, occurs under the influence of testosterone.

Endocrine abnormalities – low levels of androgens, HCG, LH, MIS

Decreased intra-abdominal pressure – prune belly syndrome, gastroschisis

RISK FACTORS

Birth prematurity is the most significant risk factor (40%).

Twins or family history (14% of boys with UDT have positive family history)

Low birth weight

CLASSIFICATION

The most useful classification for UDT is palpable (80%) vs. non-palpable.

Non-palpable include intra-abdominal and inguinal (50%), absent (20%), atrophic (30%) and sometimes ectopic testis.

Most intra-abdominal testis are close to internal inguinal ring opening.

Palpable includes true UDT and ectopic.

Ectopic Testis (< 5%)

Abnormal testis migration below the external ring of the inguinal canal (to perineum, base of penis, femoral areas)

The most common aberrant position is in the superficial inguinal pouch.

Not usually possible for ectopic testis to descend into normal position into scrotum.

Retractile Testis

An intermittent over-active cremasteric reflex causing testis to retract up and out of scrotum, which however can be manipulated down into scrotum (and stays there). [23]

Testis itself is usually normal in size and consistency.

1 / 3 can ascend and become undescended; therefore patients should be monitored in clinic as they may require future orchidopexy.

Gliding Testis

Differs from retractile testis in that manipulation down into scrotum is possible but painful, and the testis will migrate upwards again on release.

Gliding testis will only enter scrotum under tension.

It requires surgical intervention (unlike retractile testis which can be observed).

Absent Testis

Monochidism can be identified in 4% of boys with UDT (bilateral monorchidism < 1 %).

An intra-uterine gonadal vessel torsion may have led to infarction of a normal testis, a condition termed *vanishing testis syndrome*. [24]

In most cases the PPV is closed. If bilateral then patient may have raised FSH or micropenis.

DIAGNOSTIC EVALUATION

Enquire regarding risk factors such as prematurity, low birth weight, family history and maternal exposure to hormones.

Previous palpable testicle suggests testicular ascent.

Examination should evaluate:

- baby overall health, presence of other genital or constitutional abnormalities
- for palpable testicle: define the location, can it be brought down into scrotum? (painfully or pain-free)
- for non-palpable: is contralateral testis palpable? (if not, consider DSD) compensatory hypertrophy suggests affected UDT side is atrophic or absent

Imaging cannot determine with certainty that a testis is present or not (US high false-negative) and MRI is likely to require a GA anyway.

Imaging should therefore not be routinely used in further assessment for UDT.

Repeat examination should be deferred until child reaches 3 months of age.

The first step in further evaluation should include EUA, to then proceed to surgical intervention based on examination findings.

MANAGEMENT

Most testes will have descended by 3 months of age – it is unlikely that they will descend after.

BAPU suggests orchidopexy should be performed at 3–6 months of age (although 6–12 months is considered acceptable).

Any treatment leading to scrotally positioned testis should be completed by 12 months of age.

Histological examination after this age has revealed:

- Leydig cell hypoplasia
- delayed disappearance of gonocytes
- reduced number of adult dark (Ad) spermatogonia
- reduced total numbers of germ cells per testicular tubule

Earlier orchidopexy is more technically challenging (delicate vas and testicular vessels) and higher anaesthetic risk must be taken into consideration.

Reasons for correcting an UDT include:
- 10x risk of testicular cancer, therefore allowing patient to self-examine later in life (cancer risk is related to degree of UDT descent; significantly higher risk in intra-abdominal testis)
- preserve fertility (paternity rates match controls if orchidopexy performed < 2 years)
- cosmetic
- reduce the risk of torsion (UDT carries a higher risk)
- abolish risk of hernia arising from PPV

Only 1–3% of boys with UDT will develop testicular cancer (however 10% of patients with testicular cancer have a history of UDT).

INGUINAL ORCHIDOPEXY

Widely used technique with a high success rate

The steps for a standard inguinal orchidopexy:
- WHO checklist, supine, prepped and draped
- EUA to confirm palpable testis in groin
- skin crease incision superior and lateral to pubic tubercle
- open the external oblique to enter the inguinal canal and identify testis
- divide gubernaculum
- mobilise vas and vessels away from processus vaginalis (which is transfixed and divided at internal ring) and gain length by this mobilisation
- create dartos pouch in scrotum and pass the testis into this
- close both wounds and instil local anaesthetic

Informed consent must include failure to bring down, testis removal or atrophy, further surgery.

NON-PALPABLE TESTIS MANAGEMENT

Requires treatment decisions that will be made in theatre depending on findings of EUA.

If the testis is now palpable in groin on EUA, patient proceeds to inguinal orchidopexy.

If testis is not palpable, immediate laparoscopy performed to assess for intra-abdominal testis.

If testis is located within the abdominal cavity:

- if close to inguinal ring, may be possible to achieve single-stage orchidopexy
- higher testis requires two-stage Fowler-Stephens (1st stage divides testicular artery allowing growth of artery to vas from inferior vesical artery, 2nd stage brings testis into scrotum) – quote 20% risk of loss of testicle [25]
- if vessels are blind ending or end in poor nubbin of tissue, orchidectomy recommended with contra-lateral testicular fixation (risk of torsion due to possible ipsilateral vanishing testis due to intra-uterine torsion)

To check whether adequate length has been achieved, draw the testis and cord to the contralateral deep inguinal ring.

Note laparoscopy is not used to repair ipsilateral inguinal hernia or PPV if found intra-operatively.

Figure 2 – EAU 2020 algorithm for unilateral non-palpable UDT [2]

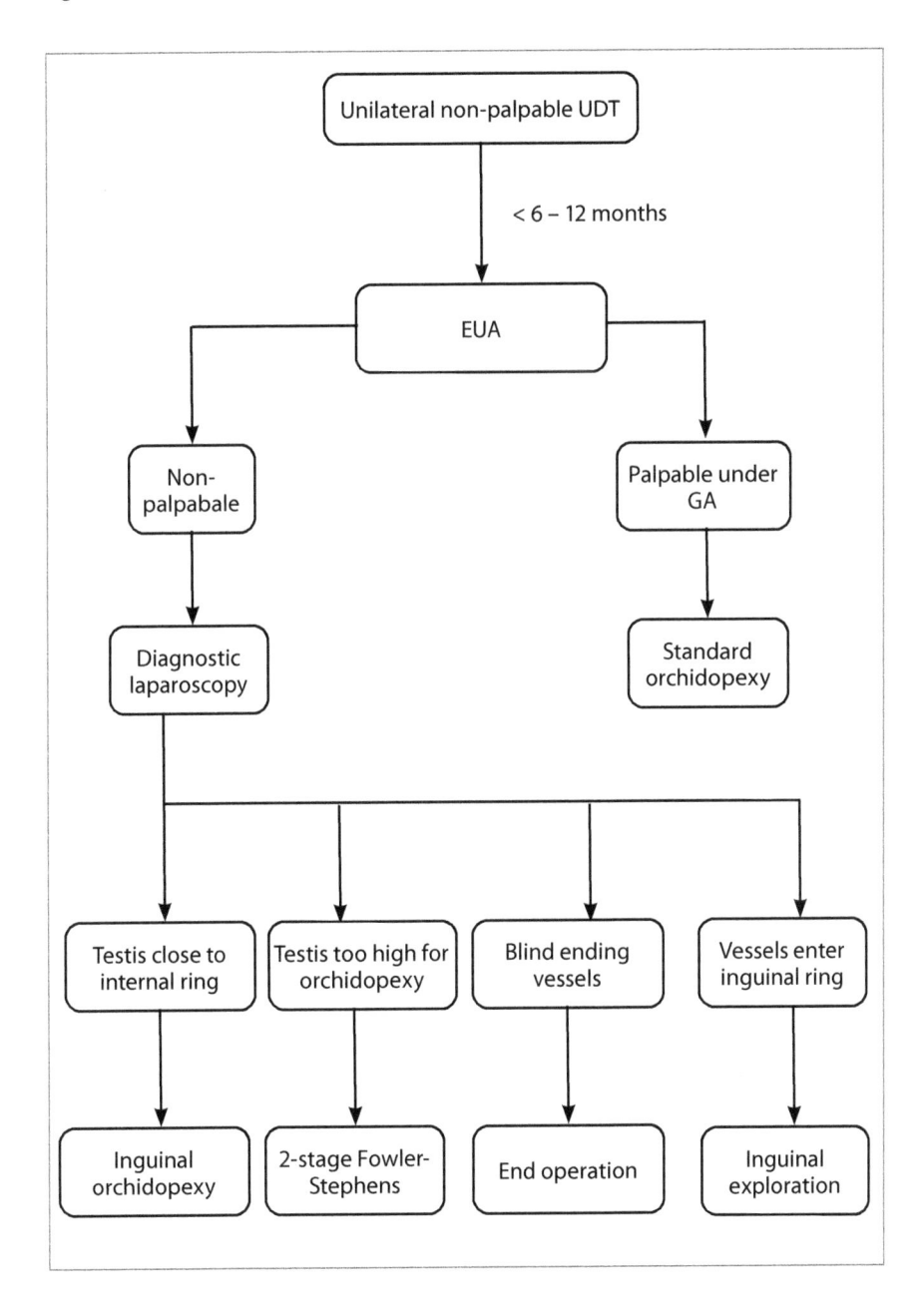

MANAGEMENT OF OLDER PATIENTS

Patients with UDT will occasionally present later in life.

Pre-pubertal management:

- < 10 years and / or bilateral UDT – proceed to bilateral orchidopexy
- > 10 years and normal contra-lateral testis – proceed to orchidectomy

Post-pubertal management:

- < 32 years and normal contra-lateral testis – proceed to orchidectomy
- > 32 years and unilateral UDT – observe and self-examine (offer orchidectomy if self-examination is difficult)

HYPOSPADIAS

EPIDEMIOLOGY

Congenital abnormality found in 1 / 250 live male births (2nd most common congenital birth defect in the male reproductive system)

7% risk in offspring of affected male, 14% risk in male siblings [26]

Higher risk in low birth weight babies

Often associated with hooded foreskin and chordee

CLASSIFICATION

Typically described in relation to the position of the urethral meatus: [27]

- *distal*, (anterior) meatus situated on glans or corona (most common 80%)
- *intermediate*, meatus on distal- or mid- penile shaft (10%)
- *proximal*, (posterior) meatus on proximal shaft, scrotum or perineum (10%)

This classification however has limited use in characterising condition's severity and indeed predicting those patients who would benefit from surgery.

Other factors are relevant such as chordee, micropenis, urethral plate quality.

AETIOLOGY

Hypospadias is a congenital deformity whereby the urethral meatus opening is abnormally sited on the ventral side of the penis.

Results from incomplete closure of urethral folds on the underside of the penis during development.

Defect in production / metabolism of foetal androgens or abnormality in tissue androgen receptors.

Chordee, arises due to abnormal urethral plate development or intrinsic corpora cavernosa abnormality.

Hooded foreskin, results from failed fusion of preputial folds.

ASSOCIATED ABNORMALITIES

Diagnostic evaluation also includes assessment of associated abnormalities, including: [2]

- UDT / cryptorchidism (10%)
- PPV or inguinal hernia (10%)

Severe hypospadias with uni- or bi-laterally impalpable testis, warrants assessment for disorders of sexual differentiation (i.e. chromosomal karyotyping).

Incidence of upper tract abnormalities is comparable to that of general population.

DIAGNOSTIC EVALUATION

The descriptive evaluation of hypospadias should include the following factors:

- presence of hooded foreskin
- curvature of penis on erection
- size of the penis
- position, shape and width of urethral opening
- presence of bilateral palpable testes

MANAGEMENT

A hypospadias does not mandate a surgical correction.

The indications for surgery focus on voiding, future sexual function and cosmetic factors, age of surgery is usually 6–18 months.

Cornerstone principles of surgery include:

- correcting any curvature (orthoplasty)
- dealing with hooded foreskin
- re-siting urethral meatus

Age at surgery for primary hypospadias repair is 6–18 months, balancing anaesthetic risk, size of penis and compliance with post-operative catheter and dressings.

Haemostasis should be meticulous and achieved by bipolar diathermy.

Sutures should be fine (6′0 or 7′0) and hence magnification lenses recommended.

Difficulty of catheter placement is most commonly due to enlargement of the utricle.

There are many different types of hypospadias repair – choice will depend on surgeon experience.

Pre-operative Hormones

Local or parenteral administration of testosterone, dihydrotestosterone or Beta-HCG is an option to enlarge glans and shaft of penis.

This may be indicated in proximal hypospadias, small penis and reduced glans circumference. [28]

CORRECTION OF CURVATURE

Functionally probably the most important aspect of the operation.

Often due to the ventral skin being too short, which is corrected by degloving the penis and excising tissue on ventral aspect (1st step in most cases which may be sufficient).

Residual curvature is due to corporal disproportion and requires straightening by dorsal plication (similar to Nesbit procedure).

Curvatures < 30° can be straightened by single dorsal plication without apparent penile shortening.

Urethral plate transection and / or ventral corporal grafting surgery are reserved for patients with curvature > 30° after de-gloving.

DEALING WITH HOODED FORESKIN

Hooded foreskin may be used as a source of dartos layer, free graft or correcting skin layer curvature.

Residual foreskin is excised to achieve circumcised appearance, although it can be preserved for foreskin reconstruction if this is the parental preference.

RE-SITING URETHRAL MEATUS

Meatal Advancement Glansplasty Incorporated (MAGPI)

Distal hypospadias only (limited to glans only)

Lateral incisions and wrap-around

Tubularisation

Involves use of urethral plate to form tube.

Tubularised Incised Plate (Snodgrass) is the most commonly performed hypospadias procedure.

The penis is de-gloved, glans wings incised to separate them from urethral plate which is incised in the midline to widen it and allow tubularisation (dartos pedicle used to cover) over catheter.

Most common cause of meatal stenosis after Snodgrass repair is suturing the urethral plate too distally.

Two-stage repair may be required for proximal cases, using buccal or preputial mucosa over a catheter (in situ for 7 days). 2nd stage tubularisation of neo-urethra is delayed for 6 months.

COMPLICATIONS

Early – bleeding, infection, dehiscence

Late – fistula (most common), meatal stenosis, urethral stricture or diverticulum, psychological [29]

Complication rates are closely correlated to surgeon case volume.

Complications are more likely to occur in distal repairs vs. proximal, and in re-do repairs (>20%).

For fistulas, management includes initially replacement of catheter and referral to Tertiary Centre for re-do surgery (≤50% recurrence).

PAEDIATRIC HYDROCOELE

Hydrocoele defined as collection of fluid between parietal and visceral layers of tunica vaginalis.

Primary hydrocoele (communicating) – based on patency of processus vaginalis

Secondary hydrocoele (non-communicating) – reactive collection by infection /trauma / tumour etc.

PRIMARY HYDROCOELE

An open PPV will allow communication with the peritoneal cavity and thus fluid transmission and the possibility of an inguinal hernia.

The size and presence of hydrocoele may thus depend on the ambulation of the patient.

The exact time of spontaneous PPV closure is not known.

90% of hydrocoeles will resolve by 12 months of age and do not require surgery.

SECONDARY HYDROCOELE

Non-communicating hydrocoeles are based on an imbalance between secretion and reabsorption of fluid, secondary to trauma, torsion or infection.

Hydrocoele of the Cord

If PPV obliterates with patency of mid-portion, a hydrocoele of the cord occurs. This is fixed in line with the cord, the testis is separate (you can get above testis on examination).

Idiopathic Scrotal Oedema

Presents as painless hemi-scrotal swelling often extending into perineum and inguinal area.

Peak incidence age 6–7 years

Warrants sonographic evaluation to rule out hydrocoele. Treated conservatively +/- NSAIDs.

DIAGNOSTIC EVALUATION

History of the swelling to include:

- age of onset
- related symptoms such as pain, inflammation, change in nappies,
- variation with position or ambulation

Examination of the abdomen and scrotum:

- if unable to get above swelling – consider inguinal hernia, communicating hydrocoele
- if able to get above swelling – consider hydrocoele of cord, testicular tumour
- transillumination – suggests hydrocoele (although intestines and tumours can transilluminate)

US +/- Doppler is best imaging with almost 100% sensitivity.

MANAGEMENT

In most boys surgical treatment of hydrocoele is not indicated within the first 12 months of life as most will resolve by this time. [30]

There is little risk with conservative management as progression to herniation is rare and does not result in incarceration (i.e. safe to wait until > 2 years of age).

If concurrent inguinal hernia is identified at presentation then surgical fixation is warranted. [31]

Herniotomy / Ligation of PPV

Identify PPV in inguinal canal and mobilise vas and testicular vessels away from this.

Ligate and divide processus vaginalis close to internal inguinal ring.

DAY-TIME LOWER URINARY TRACT CONDITIONS

Day-time LUT conditions are those presenting with LUTS including urgency, incontinence, weak stream, hesitancy, frequency.

The term is used to group functional incontinence problems in children, developed by the ICCS. [32]

Uropathy and / or neuropathy must be ruled out prior to labelling a child as having LUT condition.

Night-time wetting is known as "enuresis" – if this is the only symptom present in the child, this is termed "mono-symptomatic nocturnal enuresis".

Normal day-time control of bladder function matures 2–3 years, night-time control 3–7 years.

Frequency of voiding is 20x / day 0–12 months, decreasing to 10x / day over ensuing years and at age 7 years it is approximately 7x / day.

CLASSIFICATION

LUT conditions arise from incomplete or delayed maturation of bladder sphincter complex.

The two main groups of LUTD are:

- *filling-phase* dysfunctions, detrusor can be over- or under- active
- *voiding-phase* dysfunctions, the main cause is sphincter and pelvic floor interference during detrusor contraction (general term is *dysfunctional voiding*) weak interference ("*staccato voiding*"), strong interference (interrupted, straining)

Incontinence in children can be broadly categorised as:

- *Functional* – e.g. over-active bladder, dysfunctional voiding, vaginal reflux, giggle incontinence
- *Structural* – relating to an anatomical cause or bladder outflow obstruction, e.g. labial adhesions or masses, meatal stenosis, phimosis, posterior urethral valves, duplex kidney with abnormal moiety may suggest ectopic ureter
- *Neurogenic* – suggested if patient exhibits spinal abnormalities, peripheral neurology, severe bowel symptoms, background of known underlying neurological conditions

Dysfunctional Voiding

Involuntary external urethral sphincter contraction during voiding, resulting in a typical "staccato" voiding pattern on uroflowmetry. [33]

Treatment relies on pelvic floor relaxation and biofeedback.

Vaginal Reflux

Urine enters the vagina during voiding and then leaks out short time after when standing, characterised by incontinence following normal voiding in absence of other LUTS. [34]

Treated by getting the girl to void with widely abducted legs.

If labial adhesions are present these can be treated with topical oestrogen or surgical division.

Giggle incontinence

Incontinence triggered by laughing, this mainly affects girls who typically leak large amounts of urine (entire bladder content), however the bladder is normal between episodes.

Managed with biofeedback or in select cases with methylphenidate or oxybutynin. [35]

Pollakiuria

Disorder characterised by very high frequency of day-time micturition (up to 50x), however differentiated from OAB in that there are no night-time symptoms. [36]

Often due to significant life-event stressor, condition should resolve within 6 months.

Voiding Postponement

Children demonstrate manoeuvres to postpone voiding such as leg-crossing, squatting or Vincent's curtsy (crouching and digging heel into perineum).

Associated with behavioural or psychological problems

Over-active Bladder Syndrome

Urgency +/- urge incontinence often caused by DO.

DIAGNOSTIC EVALUATION

HISTORY

History is often the most important component of the patient evaluation and may be obtained from the parents and / or child.

The following points should be clarified in the patient history:
- *drinking habits*, enquiring regarding caffeinated or stimulant energy drinks
- *bowel habits*, enquiring about constipation (if treated can resolve LUTS) and the co-existence of bowel problems which may suggest neuropathic aetiology
- *UTIs*, enquiring about cystitis-like symptoms and reviewing MSU results
- *voiding frequency*, (best evaluated with frequency-volume chart) enquire about withholding behaviour, use of school toilets during the day
- *night-time symptoms*
- general wellbeing enquiries to include other medical conditions, developmental progress, social / domestic problems

In particular for children presenting with incontinence, the following should be defined:
- *primary vs. secondary*, were the symptoms present since birth (primary) or did child previously obtain a period of > 6 months of continence
- *incontinence pattern*, such as associated urgency, continuous (ectopic ureter), after laughing (giggle incontinence), shortly after voiding (vaginal reflux in girls)
- *severity*, both in terms of frequency of episodes and amount of urine leaked

Frequency-volume Chart

Accurate completion of FVC is mandatory for determining child's voiding frequency and volumes, and should be completed on at least two days.

(most sensibly for age > 5 years)

FVC records time / volume of each void, wetting episodes, and time / volume / type of fluid intake.

ICCS defines normal voiding frequency as 4–7x / day.

Formula to calculate bladder capacity in children < 12 years (mL) = 30 x (age in years + 1)

EXAMINATION

Thorough examination of the child should cover the following regions:

- *abdomen*, for palpable bladder, masses, or loaded bowel
- *male genitalia*, meatal opening (hypospadias) and stenosis, foreskin pathology (phimosis)
- *female genitalia*, split or bifid clitoris (epispadias), perineal excoriation due to severe wetting or vaginal reflux
- *spine*, hair patch / lipoma / pigmented lesions over midline may suggest spinal dysraphism and therefore warrants peripheral neurological examination

The examination is completed by urine dipstick testing and blood pressure recording.

IMAGING

US urinary tract may be indicated in select cases and the following findings may be relevant:

- thickened bladder with upper tract dilation, suggesting BOO
- post-void residual > 20ml is significant
- duplex kidney with abnormal upper moiety, may suggest ectopic ureter

MANAGEMENT

The mainstay of LUT conditions treatment in children involves "urotherapy", which is a broad field of non-medical / non-surgical strategies. [2]

Address constipation first since bowel problems will perpetuate bladder symptoms.

Urotherapy can be divided into "standard therapy" and "specific interventions".

Standard Therapy

Non-surgical, non-pharmacological treatment for LUT conditions.

Large part of this involves education of parent and child:
- information about normal bladder function
- ensuring correct voiding posture
- advice regarding fluid intake, limiting evening fluids, emptying before bedtime

Specific Interventions

Address particular components of the LUT conditions:

> Over-active bladder → oxybutynin 2.5–5mg BD, TENS neuromodulation
>
> Giggle incontinence → oxybutynin 2.5–5mg BD
>
> Nocturnal enuresis → pad and alarm system, desmopressin [see "Monosymptomatic Nocturnal Enuresis" station]

VUDS not routinely recommended in management of LUT conditions in children.

UDS may be considered if neuropathic pathology suspected, all treatment strategies have failed or if a diagnosis has not been made by other means. [37]

Bladder pressures consistently > 40cm H_2O may start to jeopardise the upper urinary tract.

MONOSYMPTOMATIC NOCTURNAL ENURESIS

MNE is defined as night-time incontinence in children without other LUTS and without a history of bladder dysfunction.

Primary MNE refers to children who have never been dry at night for more than 6-month period.

Secondary MNE refers to the emergence of bed-wetting after a period > 6 months of being dry.

Non-MNE includes children with associated voiding dysfunction.

EPIDEMIOLOGY

One of the most prevalent conditions in childhood

5–10% of 7 year old children have MNE. [38]

Expect a yearly resolution rate of 15%, however 7% of children wetting the bed at age 7 years, will continue to have enuresis into adulthood. [39]

More common in boys

PATHOPHYSIOLOGY

Three main factors contribute to produce nocturnal enuresis:

- *Kidneys* – high night-time urine output occurs if ADH secretion is reduced (nocturnal polyuria), the normal circadian reduction in urine output during sleep is diminished
- *Brain* – altered sleep / arousal mechanism in response to full bladder (parents report difficulty in waking child at the time of bedwetting)
- *Bladder* – reduced functional bladder capacity +/- DO

Family history, psychological factors, constipation and rUTI may also contribute.

Genetically, loci have been described on chromosomes 12, 13 and 22.

DIAGNOSTIC EVALUATION

Diagnosis is usually clinched by detailed history-taking, as clinical examination in patients with MNE is often unremarkable.

HISTORY

The following aspects should be covered during the history:
- primary or secondary MNE
- presence of day-time LUTS including day-time incontinence
- frequency, character and impact of the episodes
- family history of enuresis

EXAMINATION

Physical examination of a child with MNE is usually normal – assess the abdomen, genitalia, spine and peripheral neurology.

FVC is essential, allows evaluation of nocturnal polyuria and functional bladder capacity

Urinalysis, assessing for UTI and presence of glucose

Routine imaging is not routinely recommended for MNE but US may be used for assessment.

MANAGEMENT

Nocturnal enuresis is a stressful condition for both child and parent, which can lead to social isolation, low self-esteem and anxiety.

Treatment is advised aged > 6 years onwards, depending on the overall impact of symptoms.

Active 1st line treatments include enuresis pad and alarm system and desmopressin.

Behavioural

Emptying bladder before bedtime, reducing evening fluids, avoiding caffeinated drinks and parents waking child up at their later bedtime are all conservative strategies.

Pharmacological

Desmopressin (ADH analogue) given 200–400mcg PO before bed (nasal spray no longer advised due to risk of overdose) produces an anti-diuretic response. [40]

Success rates of 70% can be achieved.

Relapse rates are high after stopping treatment (50%) unless structured discontinuation is applied. [41]

Can be used in conjunction with oxybutynin in case of small bladder capacity, however the condition would no longer considered to be solely MNE.

Alarm Treatment

Enuresis alarm activates when the child wets to wake them up; best form for arousal disorder.

Child and parents need to persevere for weeks / months to achieve results, however success rates of 70% can be expected, with low relapse rates. [42]

URINARY TRACT INFECTIONS IN CHILDREN

EPIDEMIOLOGY

Under 12 months of age
- UTI more common in boys vs. girls
- more common in uncircumcised boys vs. circumcised

Incidence after 12 months of age of UTI is greater in girls (3%) compared to boys (1%).

The most common bacterium found in community-acquired UTI is E.coli (75%).

For nosocomial UTI, other species prevalent such as klebsiella, enterobacter, pseudomonas

40% children with UTI have underlying urinary tract abnormality (of these 70% VUR / scarring).

Increased risk of finding underlying urinary tract abnormality if positive family history for VUR and febrile UTI presentation

CLASSIFICATION

There are 5 classification systems for UTI (site and severity most important in acute setting):

1. According to Site –

    lower urinary tract (cystitis) vs. upper urinary tract

2. According to episode –

    persistent, implies re-emergence of same pathogen

    recurrent, implies infection with a different pathogen (note that E.coli, may re-occur as a different serotype)

    atypical, which according to NICE 2007 applies to: [43]
    - seriously ill / septic patient
    - palpable abdominal mass
    - infection with non-E.coli pathogen
    - failure to respond to treatment with suitable antibiotics within 48 hours

3. According to severity –

    simple UTI, child may have low-grade pyrexia and feel systemically well

    severe UTI, child has fever > 39°, dehydration and systemic malaise

4. According to symptoms –

    asymptomatic bacteriuria / UTI vs. symptomatic UTI

5. According to complicating factors –

    uncomplicated, suggests UTI in a morphologically and functionally normal urinary tract, immunocompetent patient, usually eradicated with oral antibiotics

    complicated, refers to UTI in neonates, children with pyelonephritis and patients with morphologically and / or functionally abnormal urinary tract

DIAGNOSTIC EVALUATION

The history should consider the following specific aspects:
- first / multiple episodes and their treatment
- screen for known or possible abnormalities of urinary tract
- bowel dysfunction
- family / sibling history of UTI or VUR

Fever is the most common symptom of UTI in infants > 3 months.

Urine should be collected for analysis.

Plastic bag attached to genitalia is commonly used, however has high false-positive rate.

Clean catch, involves parent catching mid-urine specimen in clean container, the glans or separated labia should be cleaned prior to procedure.

Supra-pubic aspirate, is the most sensitive method to obtain uncontaminated urine sample in children.

MSU specimen is diagnostic: [2]
- if > 10^5 CFU / mL on MSU in asymptomatic patients
- if > 10^4 CFU / mL on MSU in symptomatic patients
- if > 10^3 CFU / mL on catheter urine specimen in catheterised patients
- if > 10 CFU / mL on supra-pubic urine aspirate

Urine dipstick is appealing as provides rapid result and ready to use, however:

- bacterial conversion of nitrate to nitrite takes 4 hours in bladder (infants void often)
- not all pathogens convert nitrate to nitrite

Positive nitrite finding does have high specificity for UTI.

IMAGING

US is the 1st line investigation – in 15% abnormalities are found.

Abnormal US and concerning clinical history warrant further imaging (usually DMSA).

NICE has specific recommendations for the paediatric imaging schedule in UTI for different age groups [Tables 2–4] and questions on this schedule are common in the FRCS (Urol).

Table 2 – NICE 2007 imaging schedule for children < 6 months [43]

Test	Responds to treatment within 48 hours	Atypical UTI	Recurrent UTI
US during acute infection	NO	YES	YES
US within 6 weeks	YES	NO	NO
DMSA 4–6 months after UTI	NO	YES	YES
MCUG	NO	YES	YES

Table 3 – NICE 2007 imaging schedule for children > 6 months and < 3 years [43]

Test	Responds to treatment within 48 hours	Atypical UTI	Recurrent UTI
US during acute infection	NO	YES	NO
US within 6 weeks	NO	NO	YES
DMSA 4–6 months after UTI	NO	YES	YES
MCUG	NO	NO	NO

Table 4 – NICE 2007 imaging schedule for children > 3 years [43]

Test	Responds to treatment within 48 hours	Atypical UTI	Recurrent UTI
US during acute infection	NO	YES	NO
US within 6 weeks	NO	NO	YES
DMSA 4–6 months after UTI	NO	NO	YES
MCUG	NO	NO	NO

MANAGEMENT

The child should be resuscitated systematically according to Airway to Exposure protocol.

Follow the sepsis-6 protocol where appropriate (be aware that paediatric baseline range of vital parameters differ between age groups).

These general considerations apply to the following age groups:

- Infants < 3 months with any UTI: IV antibiotics and paediatric referral
- Infants > 3 months with cystitis: oral antibiotics as per local guidelines
- Infants > 3 months with pyelonephritis: IV antibiotics and consider paediatric referral
- Asymptomatic bacteriuria does not require antibiotics [43]

DISORDERS OF SEXUAL DEVELOPMENT

DSD are congenital conditions in which the development of chromosomal, gonadal and / or anatomical sex is atypical.

Estimated to affect 1 in 4500 births

DSD can present diagnostically:
- *Prenatal*, based on karyotype and USS findings
- *Neonatal*, based on genital examination
- *Delayed*, based on early or late puberty

The paediatric urologist plays a major role in the neonatal presentation.

DSD management requires a dedicated multi-disciplinary team approach to include geneticists, neonatologists, paediatricians, endocrinologists, gynaecologists, psychologists.

Gender assignment should not be rushed until definitive diagnosis is made. Urgent child naming is not encouraged. Registry offices allow for delays in child registration in these circumstances.

DSD is divided into the following categories:
- sex-chromosome DSD
- 46XY DSD
- 46XX DSD

EVALUATION

Detailed history should be taken to enquire: [2]
- parental consanguinity
- sibling DSD / abnormal genitalia / deaths
- FTT of the neonate
- maternal exposure to drugs (steroids, contraceptives)

Examination should include assessment of: [2]
- phallus and its length
- palpable gonads (which would be almost certainly testis, excluding 46XX DSD)
- number and location of openings in perineum (e.g. hypospadias)
- fusion of labio-scrotal folds, hymenal ring

Micropenis

Micropenis is a small but otherwise normally formed penis with a stretched length < 2cm. [44]

The penis is stretched and measured on dorsal aspect from the pubic symphysis to the glans tip. The scrotum may be underdeveloped and testes palpable but small.

Karyotyping is mandatory, endocrine assessment (LH, FSH, testosterone) and referral to paediatric endocrinologist advised.

Consider central causes (hypothalamic / pituitary) vs. testicular.

In proven androgen sensitivity, androgen therapy is recommended.

SEX CHROMOSOME DSD

These are disorders of gonadal differentiation and development, usually due to absent or disordered genetic material.

Typically occurs during meiosis (1 or 2) due to non-disjunction. Failure of separation leads to one gamete with 22 chromosomes and one with 24 (pure 45 X and 47 XXY karyotypes).

Mosaicism results from non-disjunction during mitosis at blastocyst stage (note that dysgenetic gonads are at significant higher risk of subsequent malignancy).

KLINEFELTER'S SYNDROME (47 XXY)

One of the most common chromosomal disorders (1:1000 male births), diagnosed by karyotype [45]

Underlying mechanism involves at least one extra X chromosome in addition to Y chromosome such that total chromosome number is 47+

47 XXY (occasionally 48XXXY, 49XXXXY or 46XY/47XXY mosaicism) occasionally translocation of SRY gene onto X chromosome results in 46 XX maleness syndrome – similar to Klinefelter's

Typical features include: [46]
- gynaecomastia, female fat distribution, absent facial hair
- small firm testes, azoospermia
- elevated FSH/LH, testosterone is low in 50%;
- usually infertile

Phenotype more pronounced proportional to number of X chromosomes

Presence of sperm suggests mosaicism.

8x risk of breast cancer vs. normal males; also increased risk of Leydig and Sertoli cell tumours

Klinefelter's cannot be cured however a number of treatments may help:
- testosterone replacement
- reduction mammoplasty for gynaecomastia (and risk of breast cancer)
- surveillance for breast and testicular malignancy

TURNER'S SYNDROME

Incidence 1:2500

Chromosomal abnormality in which all or part of one of the X-chromosomes is missing or altered

45 X female (occasionally 45X/46XX mosaicism; rarely 45X/46XY but important as high risk of virilisation and gonadoblastoma)

Phenotypic features: female sex, failure of secondary sexual differentiation, streak ovaries, primary amenorrhoea, short stature, webbed neck, widespread nipples, short fourth metacarpal [47]

Associated congenital abnormalities include coarctation of aorta, bicuspid aortic valve, horseshoe kidney, renal agenesis (reduced life expectancy due to cardio-vascular conditions)

Turner's syndrome cannot be cured however a number of treatments may help:
- Excision of streak gonad in those with Y chromosome material
- Surveillance for cardiovascular and renal abnormalities

MIXED GONADAL DYSGENESIS

Typically 45X/46XY mosaicism – wide spectrum of clinical manifestations

Streak gonad one side, testis (often undescended) on other with corresponding Mullerian and Wolffian ducts, phallic enlargement but with uterus and vagina

Increased risk of gonadal tumours involving testis, (gonadoblastoma) and Wilm's tumour

Mixed gonadal dysgenesis and Wilm's tumour commonly associated with Denys-Drash syndrome (triad of ambiguous genitalia, Wilm's tumour and glomerulonephritis)

VIRILISATION OF 46XX FEMALE (46 XX DSD)

Virilisation of 46 XX female due either to foetal androgen (CAH) or excess maternal androgens (e.g. androgen-secreting tumours of ovary or adrenal)

The most common type is CAH.

CONGENITAL ADRENAL HYPERPLASIA

CAH accounts for 90% of all infants with ambiguous genitalia.

Autosomal recessive disorder due to 21-hydroxylase deficiency (95% of cases) [48]

Mutation of 21-hydroxylase gene on chromosome 6 (conversion to inactive CYP21A gene)

Diagnosis – elevated 17-OH-progesterone

75% of patients present with salt-wasting and 25% with simple virilisation.

Impaired hydrocortisone production, resulting in compensatory increase ACTH and testosterone, presents with "salt-losing crisis" (dehydration, low sodium) due to aldosterone deficiency.

This is neonatal emergency – requiring IV fluids to maintain blood pressure, UE check and potassium-lowering agents, mineralo- and gluco-corticoid supplementation.

INADEQUATE VIRILISATION OF 46 XY MALE (46 XY DSD)

46 XY with defects of testosterone production / metabolism resulting in varying degrees of feminisation

The most common type is CAIS.

COMPLETE ANDROGEN INSENSITIVITY SYNDROME

CAIS is caused by androgen resistance.

With relevant family history, karyotyping can be performed at birth, otherwise difficult to detect.

X-linked recessive: Mutation of androgen receptor located on long arm of chromosome X

Phenotype and external genitalia are female, however internal genitalia are rudimentary / absent.

Lower 2 / 3 blind-ending vagina. Testes may be palpable in inguinal canal. [49]

May be detected on investigation for primary amenorrhea (raised LH and testosterone).

Management includes:

- inguinal orchidectomy due to future malignancy risk
- oestrogen replacement therapy
- vaginoplasty

5α – REDUCTASE DEFICIENCY

Autosomal recessive condition (mutation of 5αR type 2 gene) [50]

Patients are born with male gonads which can be normal, ambiguous or include normal female genitalia, however only affects those with a Y-chromosome.

Virilisation will become apparent at puberty and adults never get BPH.

MISCELLANEOUS PAEDIATRIC UROLOGY

EMBRYOLOGY OF KIDNEY

In order of appearance, the embryonic kidney transitions from pro- to meso- to meta- nephros, and all these develop from the intermediate mesoderm.

The first two regress in utero, however the metanephros (forms at gestation day 28) becomes the permanent kidney.

Renal calyces and pelvis, ureter and collecting ducts arise from the ureteric bud.

Transitional zone of the prostate and bulbourethral glands arise from the urogenital sinus.

Vas, seminal vesicle, epididymis, ejaculatory ducts, bladder trigone and central zone of the prostate arise from the mesonephric (Wolffian) ducts.

By week 12, the urachus involutes to become the median umbilical ligament. [51]

PAEDIATRIC FLUIDS

Weight (kg)	Fluid Rate
Up to 10 kg	4 mL / kg / hour for the first 10 kg
10–20 kg	2 mL / kg / hour for the next 10 kg
> 20kg	1 mL / kg / hour for every kilogram over 20 kg

Estimated circulating blood volume in child – 80 mL / kg

Fluid bolus for children – 10–20 mL / kg

WILMS' TUMOUR

EPIDEMIOLOGY

Incidence 1 : 10,000 (commonest intra-abdominal tumour of childhood)

20% of all paediatric malignancies, 80% of genitourinary malignancies

Majority present < 5 years of age (75%)

Male and female equally affected, bilateral in 5%

PATHOLOGY

Wilms' tumour contains metanephric blastema, primitive renal tubular epithelium and connective tissue components (appearing grey in colour like cerebral tissue). [52]

Histological sub-types include favourable (well-differentiated) and anaplastic (poorly differentiated).

Molecular relevance is WT1 tumour suppressor gene (11p13) mutation or deletion.

DIAGNOSTIC EVALUATION

Most common presentation is palpable abdominal mass (90%).

Other symptoms include visible haematuria (50%), hypertension (50%) and abdominal pain.

Associated syndromes include Denys-Drash (ambiguous genitalia), Beckwith-Wiedemann (macroglossia) and horseshoe kidney. [53]

1st line imaging investigation is US abdomen – upon finding a mass, patient would require standard CT thorax / abdomen / pelvis for completion staging.

Needle biopsy is recommended.

MANAGEMENT

Biopsy confirmation → neo-adjuvant chemotherapy → surgical excision → (?) adjuvant chemotherapy

Tri-modal approach to therapy: nephrectomy, vincristine / doxorubicin chemotherapy and radiotherapy

Staging [54]

Stage 1 – tumour limited to kidney, no capsular invasion, completely excised

Stage 2 – tumour outside kidney but completely removed

Stage 3 – intra-abdominal / peritoneal / IVC involvement

Stage 4 – haematogenous / extra-abdominal lymph node involvement

Stage 5 – bilateral tumours

RHABDOMYOSARCOMA

Very rare tumour of mesenchyme, resembling skeletal muscle

May involve genitourinary tract, typically bladder base, prostate, para-testicular, uterus and vagina

Increased risk in Li-Fraumeni syndrome (p53 mutation)

Embryonic forms have the better prognosis (most bladder tumours are embryonal).

NEUROBLASTOMA

Tumour arising from neuro-ectoderm – 50% occur in the adrenal gland and remainder along the sympathetic chain.

Patients tend to be more symptomatic compared to Wilms' tumour.

Median age at diagnosis is 2 years.

Poor prognostic sign is deletion of short arm of chromosome 1.

MIBG scan is highly sensitive.

Patient may have proptosis due to retro-orbital metastases.

PRUNE BELLY SYNDROME

Genetic condition almost always affecting boys.

Name arises for the wrinkled skin appearance present on the abdomen, typical triad involving:

- abdominal wall defects
- cryptorchidism (often intra-abdominal) which may be bilateral, patient typically infertile
- genitourinary defects (dilated ureter and bladder, VUR, detrusor failure)

PAEDIATRIC UROLOGY MCQS

1. Which of the following statements regarding VUR is false?
   A) it is more common in Caucasian children compared to Afro-Caribbean
   B) it is more common in girls vs. boys
   C) the most common cause in females is duplication
   D) it tends to be diagnosed at a younger age in boys
   E) Grade 3 VUR is more common than Grade 1

2. At what gestational age does the urachus involute?
   A) 8 weeks
   B) 12 weeks
   C) 16 weeks
   D) 20 weeks
   E) 24 weeks

3. Regarding Wilms' tumour, on which chromosome is the WT1 gene found?
   A) 11
   B) 13
   C) 15
   D) 17
   E) 19

4. What is the most common enzyme abnormality in CAH?
   A) 21-hydroxylase deficiency
   B) 11ß-hydroxylase deficiency
   C) 17α-hydroxylase deficiency
   D) 3ß-hydroysteroid deficiency
   E) 17ß-hydroxylase deficiency

5. What is the most accurate incidence of horseshoe kidney?
   A) 1 / 200
   B) 1 / 400
   C) 1 / 600
   D) 1 / 800
   E) 1 / 1000

6. A 2 year old boy is successfully treated with oral antibiotics only for a klebsiella UTI and discharged. Which statement regarding his follow up imaging is correct?
   A) he should have an US urinary tract within 4–6 weeks
   B) he should have an MCUG
   C) an US urinary tract at diagnosis is not required
   D) he should have a DMSA within 4–6 weeks
   E) none of the above

7. Which of the following is not a risk factor for developing hypospadias?
   A) maternal use of iron supplements
   B) paternal exposure to pesticides
   C) increasing maternal age
   D) oral contraceptive pill prior to pregnancy
   E) excess intake of phytoestrogens

8. Orchidopexy to treat UDT delayed > 12 months has been associated with all of the following histological changes except?
   A) delayed disappearance of gonocytes
   B) reduced total numbers of germ cells per testicular tubule
   C) reduced lipid quantity of Leydig cells
   D) Leydig cell hypoplasia
   E) reduced number of adult dark (Ad) spermatogonia

9. Which of the following statements regarding ectopic ureter is false?
   A) in boys the ectopic orifice is rarely below the external sphincter
   B) most common site of ectopic ureter drainage in boys is posterior urethra
   C) the upper moiety in a complete duplication tends to obstruct
   D) it is more common in girls
   E) it is less common than ureterocoele

10. A 6 year old boy is referred to you as he passes urine every 15 minutes throughout the day, but generally sleeps through the night. He does not suffer with incontinence or any other LUTS. Which of the following is the most likely diagnosis?
    A) Ochoa syndrome
    B) overactive bladder syndrome
    C) Hinman's syndrome
    D) dysfunctional voiding
    E) pollakiuria

11. Which of the following statements regarding CAIS is false?
    A) the Quigley scale uses 7 distinct classes to describe phenotypic grading
    B) the intra-abdominal gonads are testes
    C) bone mineral density is typically higher than unaffected females
    D) Leydig cell testosterone is aromatised to oestrogen
    E) Mullerian ducts automatically develop in the absence of gonadal hormones

12. Which of the following statements regarding horseshoe kidney is true?
    A) the isthmus is typically anterior to L1 – L2
    B) horseshoe kidneys are more likely to develop upper tract TCC
    C) the renal pelvis typically lies posteriorly
    D) the ascent of the kidney is typically inhibited by the superior mesenteric artery
    E) it is associated with Denys-Drash syndrome

13. An MIBG scan is used to aid in the diagnosis of which paediatric tumour?
    A) rhabdomyosarcoma
    B) neuroblastoma
    C) nephroblastoma
    D) germ cell tumour
    E) hepatoblastoma

14. A 6 week old boy born at term is referred to you as the right testis was impalpable at the 6-week baby check by the GP. Indeed, your examination confirms these findings. What is the next most appropriate step?
    A) EUA – if testis found in inguinal canal, proceed to laparoscopic right sided orchidopexy
    B) EUA – if testis is found in scrotal sac, no further operating is required
    C) EUA – if no testis is palpable, proceed to laparoscopy and 2-stage Fowler-Stephens if viable testis found in the abdomen
    D) refer for MRI
    E) no action is required at present

15. Which one of the following is not a criterion which defines an atypical UTI in children as per the NICE guidelines?
    A) poor urine flow
    B) raised creatinine
    C) abdominal mass
    D) raised white cell count
    E) Klebsiella culture

16. Which of the following statements regarding ureterocoele is false?
    A) it may be associated with either moiety of a duplex kidney
    B) it is more common in girls
    C) ectopic is more common than orthotopic ureterocoele
    D) infected obstructed ureterocoele should be managed with urgent invasive surgical decompression
    E) most ureterocoeles are associated with duplex kidneys rather than single system kidneys

17. Regarding the pharmacological therapy for MNE, which of the following statements is true?
    A) desmopressin should not be prescribed via the sublingual route
    B) fluid restriction along with desmopressin risks causing hyponatraemia
    C) immediate release is more effective than modified release oxybutynin for MNE
    D) oxybutynin is not licensed for children < 5 years of age
    E) parents should be counselled that their child may lose weight with desmopressin

18. Which of the following statements regarding PUV in males is false?
    A) vesicostomy is not known to decrease future bladder compliance and capacity
    B) type 1 category of PUV is the most common
    C) 30% of paediatric ESRF can be attributed to PUV
    D) UDT is 10x more common in patients with PUV
    E) thick-walled bladder on US is a better predictor of PUV compared to keyhole sign

19. What is the correct estimated bladder capacity for a 6 year old boy?
    A) 120mL
    B) 160mL
    C) 180mL
    D) 210mL
    E) 230mL

20. Which of the following statements regarding antibiotic prophylaxis in patients with VUR is false?
    A) the RIVUR trial did not demonstrate any protective effect of antibiotic prophylaxis against paediatric hypertension
    B) the Swedish Reflux Study showed that antibiotic prophylaxis reduced rUTI in boys but did not protect against renal scarring
    C) nitrofurantoin should not be used in children for prophylaxis if GFR < 45mL / minute
    D) cefalexin is not licensed for the prophylaxis of rUTI in children
    E) the Swedish reflux study subjected its paediatric to invasive MCUG at start and end of trial

21. Which of the following statements regarding UDT is true?
    A) ≤ 90% of all UDT are palpable
    B) the Prentiss manoeuvre involves dividing the inferior epigastric vessels
    C) 1 in 2 retractile testes can later ascend and become effectively undescended
    D) 1 in 2 non-palpable testes are absent
    E) Success of hormonal therapy for UDT is not correlated to location of UDT

22. Which of the following statements regarding the classification of VUR is false?
    A) the ureters are not dilated in grade 1
    B) refluxed urine reaches the renal pelvis in grade 2
    C) grade 2 VUR is more common than grade 3
    D) the grading system does not apply to direct retrograde study via cystoscopy
    E) grade 3 ureter is tortuous and deformed

23. Which is the most common type of composition of stones found in children?
    A) calcium oxalate
    B) uric acid
    C) cystine
    D) struvite
    E) calcium phosphate

24. Which of the following statements regarding paediatric hydrocoele is false?
    A) sclerosing agents use is limited due to risk of peritonitis
    B) standard repairs (e.g. Lord's) should be used for secondary paediatric hydrocoeles
    C) corrective surgery for a hydrocoele of the cord should excise the mass
    D) patient ambulation does not affect non-communicating hydrocoeles
    E) the processus vaginalis persists in ≤ 30% of newborns

25. Which of the following statements regarding prune belly syndrome is true?
    A) its eponymous name equivalent is Canavan's syndrome
    B) pulmonary hypoplasia and oligohydramnios feature in category 3 of Woodard classification
    C) single stage orchidopexy is rarely possible
    D) 1 in 3 will progress to ESRF requiring renal transplantation
    E) malrotation is the most common gastrointestinal associated abnormality

REFERENCES

1. Hindryckx A, De Catte L. (2011) Prenatal diagnosis of congenital renal and urinary tract malformations. *Facts, views & vision in ObGyn*, 3(3), 165.
2. Radmayr C, Bogaert G, Dogan HS et al. (2020) EAU Guidelines Paediatric Urology. Available at: https://uroweb.org/guideline/paediatric-urology/#3_12 [last accessed 5 June 2020].
3. Skoog SJ, Peters CA, Arant BS, et al. (2010) Pediatric vesicoureteral reflux guidelines panel summary report: clinical practice guidelines for screening siblings of children with vesicoureteral reflux and neonates/infants with prenatal hydronephrosis. *The Journal of urology*, 184(3), 1145–1151.
4. Alsaywid BS, Saleh H, Deshpande A, et al. (2010). High grade primary vesicoureteral reflux in boys: long-term results of a prospective cohort study. *The Journal of urology*, 184(4), 1598–1603.
5. Mohanan N, Colhoun E, Puri P. (2008). Renal parenchymal damage in intermediate and high grade infantile vesicoureteral reflux. *The Journal of urology*, 180(4S), 1635–1638.
6. Darge K, Riedmiller H. (2004). Current status of vesicoureteral reflux diagnosis. *World journal of urology*, 22(2), 88–95.
7. RIVUR Trial Investigators (2014). Antimicrobial prophylaxis for children with vesicoureteral reflux. *New England Journal of Medicine*, 370(25), 2367–2376.
8. Brandström P, Jodal U, Sillén U, et al. (2011). The Swedish reflux trial: review of a randomized, controlled trial in children with dilating vesicoureteral reflux. *Journal of pediatric urology*, 7(6), 594–600.
9. Abhyankar A, Taghizadeh AK (2018) Paediatric Urology. In: Viva Practice for the FRCS(Urol) and Postgraduate Urology Examinations 2nd Edition, CRS Press, London.
10. Hodges SJ, Patel B, McLorie G, et al. (2009) Posterior urethral valves. *The Scientific World Journal*, 9, 1119–1126.
11. Casella DP, Tomaszewski JJ, Ost MC, et al. (2012) Posterior urethral valves: renal failure and prenatal treatment. *International journal of nephrology*, 2012.
12. Nasir AA, Ameh EA, Abdur-Rahman, et al. (2011) Posterior urethral valve. *World journal of Pediatrics*, 7(3), 205.
13. Rittenberg MH, Hulbert WC, Snyder HM, et al. (1988) Protective factors in posterior urethral valves. *The Journal of urology*, 140(5 Part 1), 993–996.
14. Scott JES. (1985) Management of congenital posterior urethral valves. *British journal of urology*, 57(1), 71–77.
15. Sarhan O, El-Ghoneimi A, Hafez A, et al. (2010) Surgical complications of posterior urethral valve ablation: 20 years experience. *Journal of Pediatric surgery*, 45(11), 2222–2226.

16. Brown T, Mandell J, Lebowitz RL. (1987) Neonatal hydronephrosis in the era of sonography. *American Journal of Roentgenology, 148*(5), 959–963.
17. Sparks S, Viteri B, Sprague BM, et al. (2013) Evaluation of differential renal function and renographic patterns in patients with Dietl crisis. *The Journal of urology, 189*(2), 684–689.
18. Weizer AZ, Silverstein AD, Auge BK, et al. (2003) Determining the incidence of horseshoe kidney from radiographic data at a single institution. *The Journal of urology, 170*(5), 1722–1726.
19. Lippe B, Geffner ME, Dietrich RB, et al. (1988) Renal malformations in patients with Turner syndrome: imaging in 141 patients. *Pediatrics, 82*(6), 852–856.
20. Gairdner D. (1950) The fate of the foreskin: a study of circumcision. *Obstetrical & Gynecological Survey, 5*(5), 699.
21. Larke NL, Thomas SL, dos Santos Silva, I., et al. (2011) Male circumcision and penile cancer: a systematic review and meta-analysis. *Cancer causes & control, 22*(8), 1097–1110.
22. Summerton DJ, McNally J, Denny AJ, et al. (2000) Congenital megaprepuce: an emerging condition–how to recognize and treat it. *BJU international, 86*(4), 519–522.
23. Stec AA, Thomas JC, DeMarco RT, et al. (2007) Incidence of testicular ascent in boys with retractile testes. *The Journal of urology, 178*(4), 1722–1725.
24. Pirgon Ö, Dündar BN (2012). Vanishing testes: a literature review. *Journal of clinical research in pediatric endocrinology, 4*(3), 116.
25. Esposito C, Vallone G, Savanelli A, et al. (2009) Long-term outcome of laparoscopic Fowler-Stephens orchiopexy in boys with intra-abdominal testis. *The Journal of urology, 181*(4), 1851–1856.
26. Duckett JW, (1989) Hypospadias. *Pediatr Rev, 11*(2), 37–42.
27. Orkiszewski M. (2012) A standardized classification of hypospadias. *Journal of pediatric urology, 8*(4), 410–414.
28. Netto JMB, Ferrarez CEP, Leal AAS, et al. (2013). Hormone therapy in hypospadias surgery: a systematic review. *Journal of pediatric urology, 9*(6), 971–979.
29. Shanberg AM, Sanderson K, Duel B, (2001) Re-operative hypospadias repair using the Snodgrass incised plate urethroplasty. *BJU international, 87*(6), 544–547.
30. Koski ME, Makari JH, Adams MC, et al. (2010) Infant communicating hydroceles—do they need immediate repair or might some clinically resolve? *Journal of pediatric surgery, 45*(3), 590–593.
31. Stylianos S, Jacir NN, Harris BH, (1993). Incarceration of inguinal hernia in infants prior to elective repair. *Journal of pediatric surgery, 28*(4), 582–583.

32. Austin PF, Bauer SB, Bower W, et al. (2014) The standardization of terminology of lower urinary tract function in children and adolescents: update report from the Standardization Committee of the International Children's Continence Society. *The Journal of urology*, *191*(6), 1863–1865.
33. Yagci S, Kibar Y, Akay O, et al. (2005) The effect of biofeedback treatment on voiding and urodynamic parameters in children with voiding dysfunction. *The Journal of urology*, *174*(5), 1994–1998.
34. Kilicoglu G, Aslan AR, Oztürk M, et al. (2010) Vesicovaginal reflux: recognition and diagnosis using ultrasound. *Pediatric radiology*, *40*(1), 114.
35. Berry AK, Zderic S, Carr M. (2009) Methylphenidate for giggle incontinence. *The Journal of urology*, *182*(4), 2028–2032.
36. Watemberg N, Shalev H. (1994) Daytime urinary frequency in children. *Clinical pediatrics*, *33*(1), 50–53.
37. Hoebeke P, Bower W, Combs A, et al. (2010) Diagnostic evaluation of children with daytime incontinence. *The Journal of urology*, *183*(2), 699–703.
38. Lottmann HB, Alova I. (2007) Primary monosymptomatic nocturnal enuresis in children and adolescents. *International Journal of Clinical Practice*, *61*, 8–16.
39. Läckgren G, Hjalmås K, Gool JV, et al. (1999). Committee Report: Nocturnal enuresis: a suggestion for a European treatment strategy. *Acta paediatrica*, *88*(6), 679–690.
40. Dehoorne JL, Raes AM, Van Laecke E, et al. (2006) Desmopressin toxicity due to prolonged half-life in 18 patients with nocturnal enuresis. *The Journal of urology*, *176*(2), 754–758.
41. Gökçe Ml, Hajıyev P, Süer E, et al. (2014) Does structured withdrawal of desmopressin improve relapse rates in patients with monosymptomatic enuresis?. *The Journal of urology*, *192*(2), 530–534.
42. Glazener CM, Evans JH, Peto RE. (2005) Alarm interventions for nocturnal enuresis in children. Available at: https://www.cochranelibrary.com/cdsr/doi/10.1002/14651858.CD002911.pub2/abstract [last accessed 8 June 2020].
43. NICE Guideline: Urinary tract infection in under 16s: diagnosis and management (2007) https://www.nice.org.uk/guidance/cg54/resources/urinary-tract-infection-in-under-16s-diagnosis-and-management-pdf-975507490501 [last accessed 8 June 2020].
44. Wiygul, J, Palmer LS. (2011) Micropenis. *The Scientific World Journal*, *11*, 1462–1469.
45. Nielsen J, Wohlert M. (1991) Chromosome abnormalities found among 34910 newborn children: results from a 13-year incidence study in Århus, Denmark. *Human genetics*, *87*(1), 81–83.

46. Bojesen A, Gravholt CH. (2007). Klinefelter syndrome in clinical practice. *Nature Clinical Practice Urology*, 4(4), 192–204.
47. Stochholm K, Juul S, Juel K, et al. (2006) Prevalence, incidence, diagnostic delay, and mortality in Turner syndrome. *The Journal of Clinical Endocrinology & Metabolism*, 91(10), 3897–3902.
48. Speiser PW, White PC. (2003) Congenital adrenal hyperplasia. *New England Journal of Medicine*, 349(8), 776–788.
49. Hines M, Ahmed SF, Hughes IA. (2003) Psychological outcomes and gender-related development in complete androgen insensitivity syndrome. *Archives of sexual behavior*, 32(2), 93–101.
50. Okeigwe I, Kuohung W. (2014) 5-Alpha reductase deficiency: a 40-year retrospective review. *Current opinion in endocrinology, diabetes and obesity*, 21(6), 483–487.
51. Das JP, Vargas HA, Lee A, et al. (2020) The urachus revisited: multimodal imaging of benign & malignant urachal pathology. *The British Journal of Radiology*, 93, 20190118.
52. Kaste SC, Dome JS, Babyn PS, et al. (2008) Wilms tumour: prognostic factors, staging, therapy and late effects. *Pediatric radiology*, 38(1), 2–17.
53. Rivera MN, Haber DA. (2005) Wilms' tumour: connecting tumorigenesis and organ development in the kidney. *Nature Reviews Cancer*, 5(9), 699–712.
54. Kalapurakal JA, Dome JS, Perlman EJ, et al. (2004) Management of Wilms' tumour: current practice and future goals. *The lancet oncology*, 5(1), 37–46.

STATION 4
EMERGENCY UROLOGY

BLADDER TRAUMA

GENITAL TRAUMA

RENAL TRAUMA

URETERAL TRAUMA

URETHRAL TRAUMA

METASTATIC SPINAL CORD COMPRESSION

PENILE FRACTURE

PRIAPISM

SEPSIS, ANAPHYLAXIS AND BIOCHEMICAL EMERGENCIES

TESTICULAR TORSION

TRANS-URETHRAL RESECTION OF PROSTATE SYNDROME

URETHRAL STRICTURE

CONTENTS

BLADDER TRAUMA — **247**
- EPIDEMIOLOGY — 247
- CLASSIFICATION — 247
  - INTRA-PERITONEAL — 247
  - EXTRA-PERITONEAL — 247
- DIAGNOSTIC EVALUATION — 248
  - IMAGING — 248
- PREVENTION — 250
- MANAGEMENT — 250
  - EXTRA-PERITONEAL INJURY — 250
  - INTRA-PERITONEAL INJURY — 251
  - PENETRATING INJURY — 251
- FOLLOW-UP — 251

TESTICULAR TRAUMA — **252**
- EPIDEMIOLOGY — 252
- CLASSIFICATION — 252
- DIAGNOSTIC EVALUATION — 252
  - IMAGING — 252
- MANAGEMENT — 253

RENAL TRAUMA — **254**
- EPIDEMIOLOGY — 254
- DIAGNOSTIC EVALUATION — 254
  - IMAGING — 255
- GRADING — 255
- MANAGEMENT — 257
  - SURGICAL EXPLORATION — 258
  - PENETRATING INJURIES — 259
- FOLLOW-UP — 260

URETERAL TRAUMA — **261**
- EPIDEMIOLOGY — 261
- DIAGNOSTIC EVALUATION — 261
  - IMAGING — 262

GRADING	262
MANAGEMENT	263
SURGICAL RECONSTRUCTION	264
URETHRAL TRAUMA	**267**
EPIDEMIOLOGY	267
AETIOLOGY	267
IATROGENIC	267
ANTERIOR (NON-IATROGENIC)	268
POSTERIOR (NON-IATROGENIC)	268
DIAGNOSTIC EVALUATION	268
IMAGING	269
GRADING	270
MANAGEMENT	270
ANTERIOR URETHRAL INJURIES	270
POSTERIOR URETHRAL INJURIES	271
FEMALE URETHRAL INJURY	273
METASTATIC SPINAL CORD COMPRESSION	**274**
EPIDEMIOLOGY	274
DIAGNOSTIC EVALUATION	274
MANAGEMENT	274
PENILE FRACTURE	**276**
EPIDEMIOLOGY	276
AETIOLOGY	276
DIAGNOSTIC EVALUATION	276
IMAGING	277
MANAGEMENT	277
SURGICAL REPAIR	277
PRIAPISM	**278**
EPIDEMIOLOGY	278
PATHOPHYSIOLOGY	278
CLASSIFICATION	278
ISCHAEMIC (LOW-FLOW)	278
NON-ISCHAEMIC (HIGH-FLOW)	279

RECURRENT (STUTTERING)	279
AETIOLOGY	279
DIAGNOSTIC EVALUATION	279
PATIENT HISTORY	279
PATIENT EXAMINATION	280
BASELINE INVESTIGATIONS	280
IMAGING	280
MANAGEMENT (LOW-FLOW)	281
ASPIRATION OF CORPORA	281
INTRA-CAVERNOSAL PHENYLEPHRINE	281
SURGICAL INTERVENTION	282
PENILE PROSTHESIS INSERTION	283
MANAGEMENT (HIGH-FLOW)	283
SEPSIS, ANAPHYLAXIS AND BIOCHEMICAL EMERGENCIES	**285**
SYSTEMIC INFLAMMATORY RESPONSE SYNDROME	285
SEPSIS DEFINITIONS	285
SEPSIS-6 CARE BUNDLE PROTOCOL	286
qSOFA SCORE [8]	286
SOFA SCORE [9]	286
ANAPHYLAXIS	287
BIOCHEMICAL EMERGENCIES	287
HYPERKALAEMIA	287
HYPERCALCAEMIA	287
TESTICULAR TORSION	**289**
EPIDEMIOLOGY	289
CLASSIFICATION	289
EXTRA-VAGINAL TORSION	289
INTRA-VAGINAL TORSION	289
DIAGNOSTIC EVALUATION	289
IMAGING	290
MANAGEMENT	290
IMPACT ON FERTILITY	291
TUR SYNDROME	**292**

EPIDEMIOLOGY	292
AETIOLOGY	292
1. DILUTIONAL HYPO-NATRAEMIA	292
2. FLUID OVERLOAD	293
3. GLYCINE TOXICITY	293
MANAGEMENT	293
PREVENTION	293
RECOGNITION	294
TREATMENT	294
COMPONENTS OF COMMON IV FLUIDS:	295
URETHRAL STRICTURES	**296**
AETIOLOGY	296
DIAGNOSTIC EVALUATION	296
MANAGEMENT	297
SHORT STRICTURES	297
DE-NOVO SHORT STRICTURES	298
LONG STRICTURES	298
BUCCAL MUCOSA	298
REFERENCES	**300**
EMERGENCY UROLOGY MCQS	**301**

BLADDER TRAUMA

EPIDEMIOLOGY

Bladder is urological organ that most often suffers iatrogenic bladder injury – the most common procedure causing perforation is TURBT.

Risk factors include old age, female gender, large tumour and tumour location on dome.

Iatrogenic bladder injury can be internal (cystoscopic) or external (laparoscopy or open surgery).

RTAs most common cause of blunt bladder injury, followed by industrial trauma and falls.

60–90% of blunt trauma have associated pelvic fractures.

Pelvic fractures are associated with bladder injury in 5% of cases, and a combination of bladder and urethral injuries are noted in < 20%.

CLASSIFICATION

Bladder ruptures can be considered:

- *intra-peritoneal* (IPR) (30%) or *extra-peritoneal* (EPR) (50%)
- bladder contusion
- combined intra- and extra- peritoneal rupture

INTRA-PERITONEAL

The peritoneum overlying the bladder is breached allowing urine to escape into peritoneal cavity.

Ruptures tend to occur due to sudden rise in intra-vesical pressure (eg. Direct blow to distended bladder) and the dome is the weakest point where rupture is most likely to occur.

Clinical signs include low return of irrigation fluid, abdominal distension and bladder not filling.

EXTRA-PERITONEAL

Pelvic fractures are almost always associated with extra-peritoneal fractures.

Injury usually caused by distortion of pelvic ring and shearing of anterolateral bladder wall near the bladder base at the fascial attachments.

DIAGNOSTIC EVALUATION

The principal sign of bladder injury is visible haematuria.

Classic triad for bladder perforation:

- lower abdominal pain, inability to void and visible haematuria

Bladder injury may be detected cystoscopicallly directly at the time of injury – a dark hole is seen with bowel on the other side – no further imaging required.

For laparoscopic or open surgical injuries, urine may contaminate the operative field, and blood or gas may enter the catheter bag.

Pelvic fracture + visible haematuria = absolute indication for further imaging

Displacement of pelvic ring > 1cm + non-visible haematuria = further imaging indicated

Abdominal distension may occur in context of urinary ascites, UEs will show rise in urea and creatinine due to re-absorption of of urea nitrogen and creatinine.

IMAGING

The preferred imaging modality to detect non-iatrogenic bladder injury or suspected iatrogenic bladder injury post-operatively is cystography.

Cystoscopy is the preferred method for detecting intra-operative bladder injuries.

(Stress) Cystography

Requires catheterisation (be aware of potential urethral trauma)

Must be performed with > 300 mL of water-soluble contrast, in order to distend the bladder and adequately diagnose perforation

(For children, 60mL + 30mL for every year of age up to 400mL total)

Sub-filled bladder may result in clot / omentum / bowel loop plugging a perforation.

Antero-posterior and post-drainage films are taken.

IPR reveals contrast in or throughout peritoneal cavity highlighting bowel loops (CT may even reveal contrast around the liver).

EPR will reveal flame-shaped areas of extravasation in peri-vesical soft tissues.

Plain and CT cystography have comparable sensitivity (95%) and specificity (100%).

CT cystography (300mL of contrast into bladder via catheter and CT of pelvis) is superior at identifying bony fragments and can detect other abdominal injuries.

Cystoscopy

Allows accurate localisation of bladder injury in relation to trigone and ureteric orifices.

A bladder that does not fill despite irrigation suggests large perforation, the surgeon must also palpate the abdomen for distension due to irrigation fluid in peritoneal cavity.

CT urogram is not adequate as the bladder is a compliant organ and the amount of contrast in bladder would be insufficient to reliably diagnose perforation.

AAST Bladder Injury Scale

Table 1 – The AAST's bladder trauma scale [1]

Grade	Description of Injury
I	*Haematoma* (contusion) and / or partial thickness *laceration*
II	*Laceration* – extra-peritoneal bladder wall < 2 cm
III	*Laceration* – extra-peritoneal (≥ 2cm) or intra-peritoneal bladder wall (< 2cm)
IV	*Laceration* – intra-peritoneal bladder wall (≥ 2cm)
V	*Laceration* – intra-or extra-peritoneal bladder wall extending to bladder neck, trigone or ureteric orifices

PREVENTION

The following strategies can be employed to reduce the risk of intra-operative bladder wall perforation during procedures involving cystoscopic resection:

- give general anaesthesia with muscle paralysis
- reduce current on diathermy settings
- small, short controlled swipes with the diathermy loop
- keep the bladder under-filled during cystoscopy
- obturator nerve block

For abdominal procedures carrying a significant risk of bladder injury, insert catheter at start.

MANAGEMENT

For trauma cases initial management adopts systematic Airway to Exposure assessment of the patient, adhering to ATLS principles with a multi-disciplinary approach.

Resuscitation should include administration of broad-spectrum antibiotics as per local guidelines.

EXTRA-PERITONEAL INJURY

Most EPRs do not require surgical repair and can be managed conservatively:

- broad-spectrum antibiotics
- close observation of vital parameters
- urethral catheter on free drainage for > 10 days followed by repeat cystography

EPRs may be repaired when there are other concomitant injuries that necessitate abdomino-pelvic surgery anyway e.g. pelvic bone fragments, recto-vaginal injuries.

This is to reduce the risk of infective complications.

Repair is 2-layer closure with 2'0 vicryl (absorbable) sutures.

Persisting extravasation (i.e. failure to heal) may also warrant surgical repair of EPR.

INTRA-PERITONEAL INJURY

IPRs should always be managed by formal surgical repair, as intra-peritoneal urine extravasation can lead to peritonitis and become life-threatening.

This is performed by lower midline laparotomy and double-layer closure with absorbable sutures.

Catheter should be inserted and cystography performed after > 10 days.

IPR can be managed conservatively if small and delayed recognition after surgery, when the patient is clinically well and no signs of fever or peritonitis.

PENETRATING INJURY

Bladder rupture due to penetrating injury mandates emergency surgical exploration.

The entirety of bladder wall and ureteric orifices must be inspected and primary closure advised.

FOLLOW-UP

Continuous bladder catheter drainage required to keep the intra-vesical pressure low.

Repeat cystography is recommended > 10 days after injury. If this shows ongoing extravasation, catheter should again be left on free drainage and scan repeated in 7 days.

TESTICULAR TRAUMA

EPIDEMIOLOGY

Most civilian trauma is blunt injury.

More common in young males, due to anatomical differences, increased risk of RTCs and participation in contact sports.

Penetrating injury affects both testes in 30% (blunt trauma is bilateral in 1%) and are also associated with other concomitant injuries in 70%.

CLASSIFICATION

Haematocoele, occurs when bleeding is confined within the tunica vaginalis.

Intra-parenchymal (intra-testicular) bleeding occurs within the testis itself.

Testicular dislocation implies re-positioning of the testis within superficial inguinal ring, the inguinal canal or abdominal cavity.

Testicular rupture implies disruption of the tunica albuginea.

DIAGNOSTIC EVALUATION

Patient *history* should address specifically:
- mechanism / time of injury
- presence and evolvement of pain / swelling
- infective risk factors for penetrating injuries

Patient *examination* should assess specifically:
- whether testes are palpable, tender, smooth and intact
- degree of scrotal swelling (quantify size and compare to contralateral testis)

IMAGING

Scrotal US is the diagnostic imaging modality of choice for assessing scrotal trauma.

Primary aim of US is to detect integrity of tunica albuginea (specificity 75%, specificity 64%) and vascularity of testis.

Heterogenecity within testis on US suggests an intra-testicular bleed may have occurred.

MANAGEMENT

Trauma patients should be resuscitated systematically in an Airway to Exposure sequence, adhering to ATLS principles and adopting a multi-disciplinary management strategy.

Penetrating trauma should undergo urgent scrotal exploration, washout and debridement of non-viable tissue. Tetanus prophylaxis is mandatory along with prophylactic antibiotics.

Haematocoeles should be managed clinically and according to size, the concern relating to the raised pressure within the scrotum that can lead to testicular ischaemia.

Smaller haematocoeles can be managed conservatively with ice, elevation and rest.

Consider operative drainage if affected hemi-scrotum is > 3x size of the contra-lateral testis.

Orchidectomy rates are higher in patients undergoing delayed (80%) vs. early (< 3 days) (30%) surgical intervention.

Testicular rupture should be taken urgently to theatre for exploration, the tunica albuginea can be closed with 4'0 absorbable sutures if the testis is viable e.g. 4'0 vicryl.

Consider sperm banking in cases of severe bilateral testicular injury.

RENAL TRAUMA

EPIDEMIOLOGY

Renal trauma occurs in < 5% of all cases of major trauma (protected as retro-peritoneal structures, therefore requires considerable force and likely collateral injuries present).

Incidence is 5 per 100,000 population – higher for young men.

Vast majority of injuries in Europe are *blunt* trauma (97%) rather than *penetrating*, and most can be managed without surgical intervention.

Renal pedicle injuries are rare in blunt trauma (< 5%) and can be due to rapid deceleration injuries.

Most common cause of blunt injuries include RTCs, falls from height or sporting injuries.

Penetrating injuries are more common in urban areas, mainly involving stab or gunshot wounds to the flank, and are usually more severe than blunt injuries.

50% penetrating renal trauma and visible haematuria (VH) have Grade III or above injuries.

DIAGNOSTIC EVALUATION

Patient *history* should focus on the relevant factors:
- mechanism and time of injury
- any blood in the urine
- previous urological history
- relevant medical history to include anti-coagulation status and pre-existing renal disease

Patient *examination* should initially adhere to ATLS principles, adopting a multi-disciplinary approach liaising with A+E / orthopaedics / general surgery / anaesthetics.

Perform systematic Airway to Exposure examination. Record extent of bruising and tenderness.

Record vital signs throughout the diagnostic evaluation.

The lowest recorded systolic BP is used to determine need for renal imaging.

Urinanalysis is crucial for evaluating haematuria and thus determining need for further imaging (recall that microscopic analysis of > 5 RBCs / high power field is more reliable).

IMAGING

Spiral CT scan with contrast is the investigation of choice.

CT allows grading of injury, assessment of contra-lateral kidney and injuries to other organs.

Indications for CT scanning in a stable patient following renal trauma as per the EAU Guidelines:

- penetrating trauma
- rapid deceleration injury (or significant mechanism)
- associated systolic BP < 90 mmHg at any time
- associated visible haematuria
- associated NVH / VH in children (i.e. lower threshold for imaging)

Adults with no visible haematuria, normal BP and no significant mechanism of injury do not require routine initial CT imaging (chance of significant injury 0.2%).

Haemodynamically unstable patient may preclude CT imaging and need direct transfer to theatre.

Spiral CT is performed with initial arterial and portal-venous phases (assess vascular injuries) and delayed urographic phase after 10 minutes (assess collecting system injuries).

Trauma CT

Local protocols may vary, however an emergency trauma CT series as standard:

- non-contrast CT head and C-spine
- followed by 150mL (IV) contrast, for arterial phase (vascular injuries, 15–30s), porto-venous phase (visceral injuries, ~ 60s) and delayed phase (urothelial injuries, 5–10 minutes)

GRADING

The AAST grading system is based primarily on CT findings, and is also used UK practice:

STATION 4: EMERGENCY UROLOGY

Table 2 – The AAST's renal trauma scale [1]

Grade	Description of Injury
I	*Contusion* or non-expanding sub-capsular haematoma
	No laceration
II	Non-expanding peri-renal haematoma
	Cortical *laceration* < 1cm deep (without urinary extravasation)
III	Cortical *laceration* > 1cm deep (without urinary extravasation)
IV	*Laceration* – extending into collecting system
	Vascular – segmental renal artery / vein injury with contained haematoma, or partial vessel laceration, or vessel thrombosis
V	*Laceration* – shattered kidney
	Vascular – renal pedicle avulsion

Image 1 – AAST grading of renal trauma]

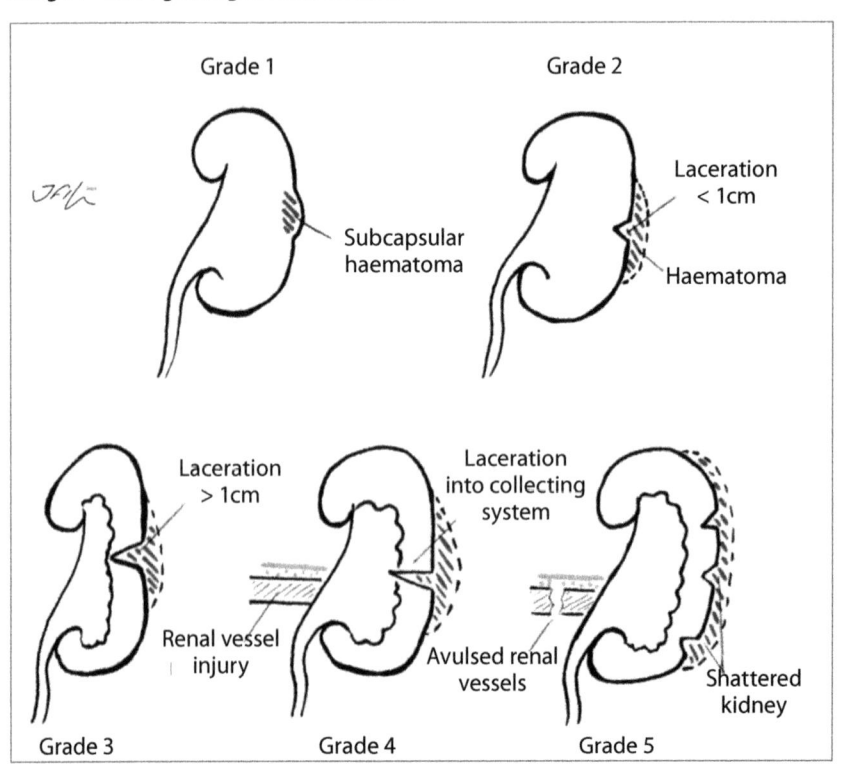

Grade 1 — Subcapsular haematoma
Grade 2 — Laceration < 1cm, Haematoma
Grade 3 — Laceration > 1cm
Grade 4 — Renal vessel injury, Laceration into collecting system, Avulsed renal vessels
Grade 5 — Shattered kidney

MANAGEMENT

Non-operative management has become the treatment of choice for most renal injuries, as it is associated with lower nephrectomy rate and no adverse impact on long term morbidity.

Operative intervention is required in < 5% of all blunt renal trauma cases.

Haemodynamic stability is the primary criterion for the management of all renal injuries.

The following common scenarios can be managed as follows:
- NVH + systolic BP > 90 mmHg = no imaging or admission required
- All Grade 1 and 2 injuries = conservative management
- Most Grade 3 injuries = conservative management

The potential complications of conservative management of renal trauma include:
- *early*, such as secondary haemorrhage, urinoma formation requiring drainage or stenting, infection and abscess formation, AV-fistula or pseudo-aneurysm formation
- *late*, such as hypertension and fibrosis (Page kidney), renal insufficiency, chronic pyelonephritis, renal artery thrombosis

High-Grade Injuries (IV and V)

Can be managed non-operatively if patient is haemodynamically stable.

Any uncontrolled bleeding will require surgical exploration – nephrectomy is indicated in most cases as Grade V injuries function poorly if repaired.

Angio-embolisation can be employed in haemodynamically stable patients, likely to be most beneficial in high grade injuries (IV and V).

Urinary Extravasation

90% of these injuries will heal spontaneously and do not require surgical exploration.

Associated bowel injuries with urinary extravasation is an indication to explore.

Monitor for fever or persisting pain (urinoma) and for significant extravasation, consider placing a ureteric stent.

SURGICAL EXPLORATION

Indications for emergency laparotomy for blunt and penetrating renal trauma include:

- persisting blood loss causing hypovolaemic shock
- renal pedicle avulsion (Grade 5 vascular injuries) but not Grade 5 parenchymal injury patients who are haemodynamically stable

During exploratory laparotomy performed for associated injuries in trauma, the decision to further explore the kidney include:

- expanding and / or pulsating retro-peritoneal haematoma
- urinary extravasation and associated bowel injury (bowel contents mixing with urine is a strong risk factor for developing over-whelming sepsis)

If the patient's clinical condition has been critical such that it has not been possible to arrange CT imaging prior to theatre, arrange one-shot on table intravenous urogram (IVU).

IVU done via injection of 2mL / kg contrast, allows assessment of two functional kidneys, extravasation on delayed portable XR, if normal may avoid need for kidney exploration.

Surgical exploration is performed as follows:

- generous midline laparotomy from sternum to pubis
- small bowel gently retracted away to expose retroperitoneum
- incise peritoneum over aorta above the inferior mesenteric artery
- superior dissection to locate the renal arteries and veins which can be ligated
- reflect the colon to expose the kidney

If at time of exploration the haematoma is found to be non-expanding and non-pulsatile, most can be left alone, as kidney exploration increases chance of resulting nephrectomy.

Surgery for Reno-vascular Injuries

Most kidneys will not function after arterial injury – reconstruction may only be indicated if diagnosed very quickly in solitary kidneys or bilateral injuries.

Renal vein injuries need to ensure the avulsion from IVC has been repaired first, the renal vein can be tied off to allow drainage from kidney via gonadal and adrenal veins.

PENETRATING INJURIES

The broad principles of management of penetrating renal injuries are similar.

Penetrating injury is an indication to undergo spiral CT scanning with contrast regardless of haematuria status, and therefore even minor grades of injury may be detected.

High grades (IV and V) are likely to require urgent surgery and renal exploration.

EAU Guidelines for Penetrating Renal Trauma [2]

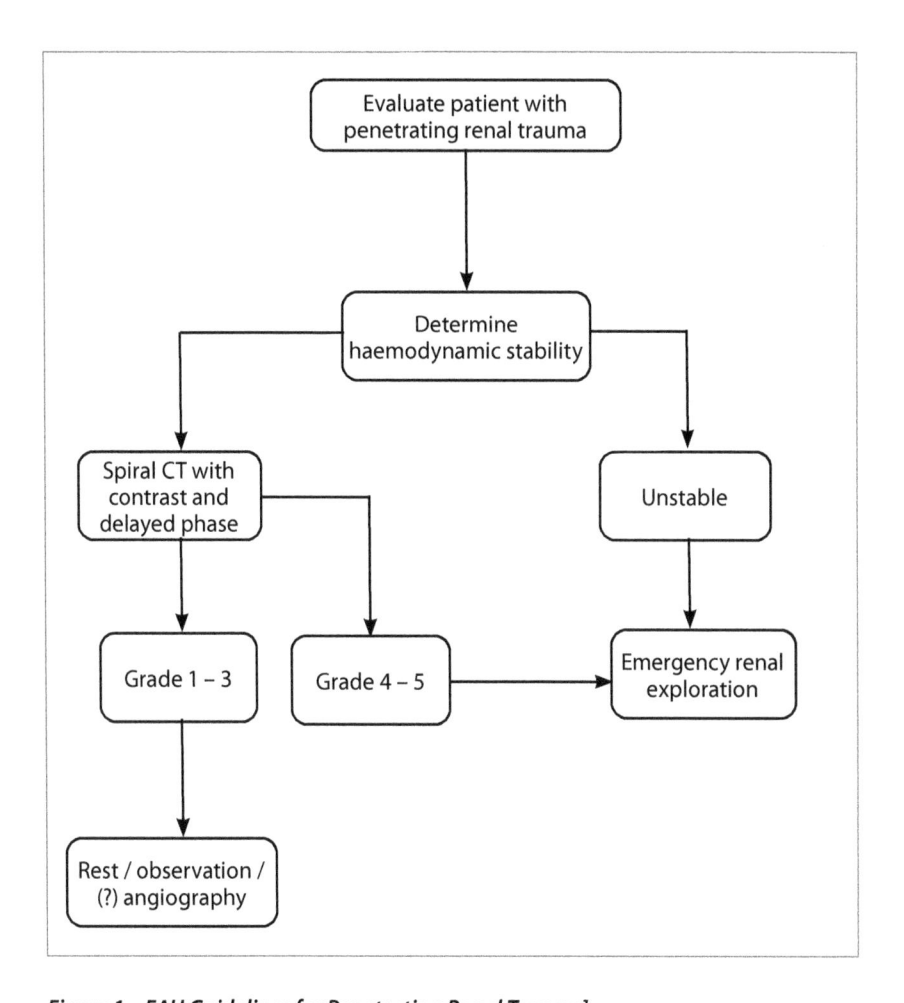

Figure 1 – EAU Guidelines for Penetrating Renal Trauma]

FOLLOW-UP

Risk of complications in conservatively treated patients increases with injury grade.

Repeat CT 2–4 days after Grade 3–5 injury should be considered, particularly if worsening flank pain, onset of fever or falling haemoglobin.

Decline in long-term renal function correlates with grade. DMSA can evaluate further.

Follow-up should include BP measurement, urinanalysis and UEs.

URETERAL TRAUMA

EPIDEMIOLOGY

Ureteric trauma accounts for < 2.5% of all trauma to urinary tract.

Iatrogenic trauma during surgery is the commonest cause (80%).

Iatrogenic injuries include suture ligation, clamp crushing, partial / complete transection, thermal injury or ischaemia from devascularation.

Gynaecological operations are the commonest cause of iatrogenic injuries to the ureter.

Routine prophylactic stenting before complex abdominal surgery is not cost-effective and does not decrease the rate of injuries.

External causes include RTCs in 1 / 3 of cases (blunt deceleration avulsing ureter from renal pelvis) and gunshot (2% of all wounds) and should be suspected in any penetrating injury.

DIAGNOSTIC EVALUATION

The injury may be suspected intra-operatively in which case it can be dealt with immediately, however often the injury will not become apparent for days / weeks after surgery.

Patient history or history from colleague should enquire regarding:
- details of surgical procedure / difficulties / indication (read operation note)
- past medical history to include abdo- / gynae- / uro – logical surgery, radiotherapy
- flank pain
- haematuria (only present in 50% of injuries)
- urinoma, suggested by fever, persistent drain output, abdominal swelling, ileus

Drain fluid (where applicable) should be tested for urea and creatinine, and should have higher creatinine than serum (drain fluid creatinine > 300 μmol / L suggests urine).

IMAGING

Post-operative Diagnosis / External Cause

CT urogram is ideal investigation, extravasation of contrast is the hallmark sign of ureteral injury.

Hydronephrosis, mild ureteral dilatation or urinoma may however be the only radiological signs.

US may show hydronephrosis, however insufficient investigation as complete transection leaks urine into peritoneal cavity with no obstruction or hydronephrosis.

For patients with a nephrostomy, antegrade nephrostogram will aid in confirming diagnosis.

Intra-operative Diagnosis

Direct, by full mobilisation of the ureter by packing bowel out the way and examining the full length (lower end if more difficult)

Retrograde ureterography, is a very accurate method via cystoscope to look for contrast extravasation and should be undertaken bilaterally.

On table IVU is technically difficult and unreliable in diagnosis.

GRADING

The AAST has defined a grading system for ureteral injuries [Table 3].

Table 3 – The AAST's ureteric trauma scale [1]

Grade of Ureteric Injury (AAST)	Injury Description	Management options
I	Haematoma only	Conservative +/- stent
II	Laceration < 50% circumference	Stent +/- suture
III	Laceration > 50% circumference	Stent +/- suture Uretero-ureterostomy +/- stent
IV	Complete tear < 2cm of devascularisation	Ureteric reconstruction
V	Complete tear > 2cm of devascularisation	Ureteric reconstruction

MANAGEMENT

Management options for ureteral trauma depend on:
- whether injury is recognised intra-operatively or delayed
- level of injury
- other associated problems (e.g. active infection, other traumatic injuries)

Intra-operatively the best time to repair a ureteric injury is as soon as it is detected, except:
- evidence of active infection at the proposed repair site
- patient unsafe for prolonged general anaesthesia

For most delayed post-operative diagnoses associated with obstructive hydronephrosis, consider nephrostomy insertion +/- ureteric stent and delaying definitive repair.

For an unstable trauma patient ➜ ligate ureter, insert nephrostomy and delay definitive repair.

Ureteric Stenting

Endo-urological treatment of ureteral injuries by stenting is the first step in most cases.

Open surgical repair is indicated in the event of failure.

Can be performed via retrograde or antegrade route.

Stent should remain in situ for minimum of 6 weeks. Patient can be listed for stent removal under GA and on-table retrograde study to ensure resolution of injury.

SURGICAL RECONSTRUCTION

Where technically possible, intra-operatively diagnosed injuries can be dealt with immediately.

For delayed diagnosed ureteric injuries, current belief is that timing of reconstructive surgery is not most important factor and can be done early, as long as the patient is clinically stable.

Proximal / Mid-ureteral Injury

For ureteral injuries < 3cm in length
- primary uretero-ureterostomy
- (alternatively if primary anastomosis not possible) uretero-calycostomy

For extensive ureteral loss, consider transuretero-ureterostomy (proximal stump of ureter is transposed across midline and anastomosed to contra-lateral ureter).

Distal Ureteral Injury

Distal injuries should undergo re-implantation as blood supply to distal ureter is jeopardised.

Psoas hitch, is reconstructive operation for more distal injuries:
- bladder is opened via surgical incision (held with two stay sutures)
- bladder pulled up by inserting index finger and is secured to the psoas muscle, to reduce distance between ipsilateral distal ureter and bladder
- the contra-lateral superior vesical pedicle is also divided to aid this manoeuvre
- uretero-neocystostomy is then performed [Image 2]

Boari flap, involves tubularisation of flap of bladder to extend from bladder to ureter, an option for ureteric reimplantation when diseased segment is long (e.g. > 5 cm) [Image 3]

The base of the flap should be broader than the tip, to reduce the risk of flap ischaemia.

URETERAL TRAUMA 265

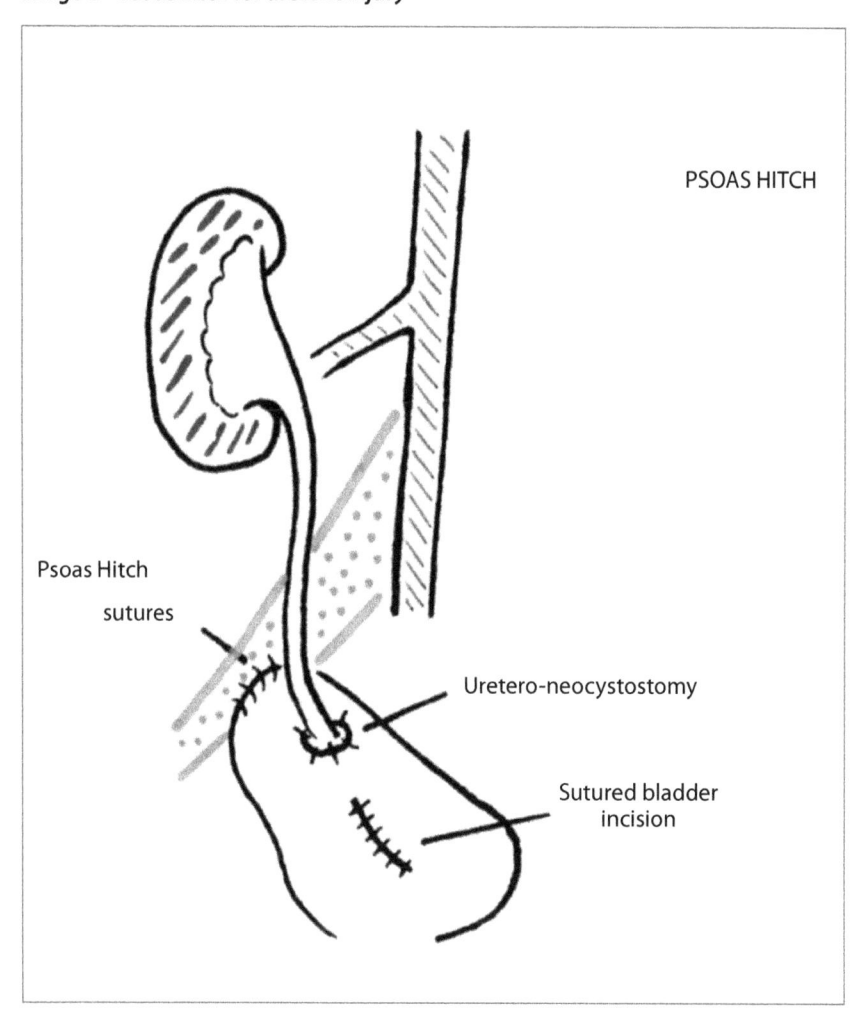

Image 2 – Psoas hitch for ureteric injury

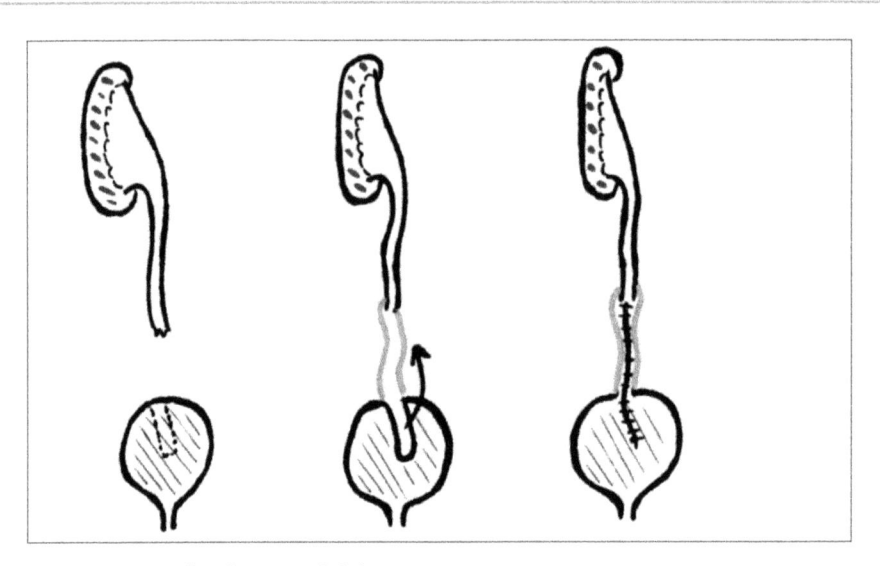

Image 3 – Boari flap for ureteric injury

Options for ureteric surgical reconstruction are summarised in [Table 4]. [3]

Table 4 – options of surgical repair for ureteric injuries divided by location of injury

Ureteric Injury Location	Option for Reconstruction
Distal ureter	Uretero-ureterostomy
	Primary re-implantation
	Psoas hitch or Boari flap
Mid-ureter	Uretero-ureterostomy
	Boari flap
	Transuretero-ureterostomy
Proximal ureter	Uretero-ureterostomy
	Uretero-calycostomy
	Transuretero-ureterostomy
Complete avulsion or injury	Ileal inter-position
	Renal auto-transplantation

Principles underpinning ureteric reconstruction are tension-free, spatulated anastomosis with fine absorbable sutures (5'0 / 6'0), placement of stent and drain.

Consider further additional protective omental interposition.

URETHRAL TRAUMA

EPIDEMIOLOGY

Most common cause of urethral trauma seen in urological practice is iatrogenic.

In anterior non-iatrogenic urethral trauma the most common cause is blunt trauma by straddle injuries.

In posterior non-iatrogenic urethral trauma almost all injuries are a consequence of pelvic fracture.

AETIOLOGY

IATROGENIC

Urethral instrumentation is by far the most common cause of urethral trauma in the Western world, and can affect all segments of the urethra.

1. Catheterisation

Most strictures caused by catheterisation affect the bulbar urethra.

Size and type of catheter have an important impact on urethral stricture formation. Smaller gauge and silicone catheters are associated with lower urethral morbidity.

Balloon inflation in the anterior urethra is also a potential cause of injury.

2. Trans-urethral surgery

Meatal strictures occur as a result of mismatch between size of instrument and meatal diameter.

Strictures may result from dispersion of electrical current, this risk can be reduced by insulation using copious amounts of lubrication.

Stricture rates for mono- and bi- polar TUR resection are comparable.

3. Radiotherapy for Prostate Cancer

Both brachytherapy and radical radiotherapy are recognised causes of urethral strictures.

4. Surgery for Prostate Cancer

Risk of urethral stricture 8% for all patients undergoing any radical treatment of prostate cancer, anastomotic strictures rates comparable for laparoscopic and robot-assisted surgeries.

Greatest risk for radical prostatectomy patients combined with EBRT.

ANTERIOR (NON-IATROGENIC)

Most common cause is straddle injury (or a kick) whereby the bulbar urethra is crushed against the pubic symphysis.

Less common causes include concomitant penile fracture, foreign body insertion into urethra and penetrating wounds (stab or gunshot).

POSTERIOR (NON-IATROGENIC)

Most injuries to the posterior urethra are related to pelvic fractures (RTCs, crush injury, falls).

Urethral injuries are not directly life-threatening, their association with pelvic fractures and / or thoraco-abdominal injuries can be.

Surgically these injuries are described as either *partial* or *complete* ruptures.

In complete ruptures there is a gap between disrupted ends of the urethra. These ends will retract and eventually fibrous tissue fills the space in-between them.

Complete rupture occurs due to shearing effect of bone disruption.

The prostate (fixed to symphysis via pubo-prostatic ligaments) moves in one direction, whilst the membranous urethra (fixed in the urogenital diaphragm) move in another.

These injuries are also called pelvic fracture posterior urethral distraction defects (PFUDD).

Delayed morbidity associated with posterior urethral injuries include stricture formation, ED and incontinence.

DIAGNOSTIC EVALUATION

Patient *history* should enquire specifically regarding:
- mechanism of injury
- passage of blood per urethra (cardinal sign of urethral injury)

- difficulty voiding (often associated with complete rupture)
- lower abdominal pain

Patient *examination* should assess specifically for:
- palpable bladder (suggesting inability to void)
- pattern of bruising to perineum, groin and abdomen (consider butterfly wing pattern)
- DRE for pelvic haematoma (soft, boggy swelling), blood on the glove (rectal injury in 5% pelvic fractures) and high-riding prostate (pushed up by haematoma)

Note that it is safe and acceptable to attempt gentle passage of a urethral catheter in the context of pelvic fracture. Any resistance should result in abandoning and inserting SPC.

Failure to insert a catheter may suggest urethral injury.

IMAGING

Retrograde urethrography (RU) is diagnostic investigation of choice for suspected urethral injury.

RU is performed with the following technique:
- 12F catheter placed in fossa navicularis
- inflate balloon to 2mL to create a seal preventing leakage of contrast
- 20–30mL of water-soluble contrast injected using fluoroscopic guidance
- optimum position is 30% oblique with hip and knee flexed (may not be possible in trauma scenario, in which case supine is adequate)
- AP films required with oblique C-arm (as bulbar urethra is superimposed on itself)

The distinction between complete and partial injury is not always clear.

Contrast extravasation on RU is pathognomic for urethral injury:
- urethral extravasation with bladder filling suggests partial rupture
- massive extravasation without bladder filling suggest complete rupture

If a SPC is in-situ, an antegrade urethrogram can be performed with contrast via the SPC.

If urethral catheter is in-situ (excludes complete rupture) pass a 6F nasogastric tube alongside the catheter and flush contrast down to exclude extravasation.

Recall that as urethra passes through pelvic floor (membranous) there is physiological narrowing, which may mimic a stricture on a RU.

GRADING

The AAST has defined a grading system for urethral injuries [Table 5].

Table 5 – The AAST's urethral trauma scale [1]

Grade	Description	Treatment options
I	Contusion	No treatment required
II	Stretch injury	Conservatively (with SPC or urethral catheter)
III	Partial disruption	Conservatively (with SPC or urethral catheter)
IV	Complete disruption	Immediate endoscopic realignment vs. delayed urethroplasty
V	Complete disruption	Immediate endoscopic realignment vs. delayed urethroplasty

MANAGEMENT

Commence with systematic Airway to Exposure patient assessment in line with ATLS principles and via a multi-disciplinary approach.

Broad spectrum antibiotics as per local guidelines should be given if urological injury suspected.

One attempt at gentle urethral catheterisation is permissible even in context of pelvic fracture.

Failed urethral catheterisation mandates SPC insertion, which may be US-guided however may require open cystostomy if bladder is collapsed.

ANTERIOR URETHRAL INJURIES

Contusions without rupture can be managed by 12F catheter insertion and removal in 7 days.

Partial ruptures can be managed with temporary urinary diversion via SPC (preferable as urethral catheter can result in complete rupture).

Repeat voiding cystogram in 2 weeks, remove SPC if normal (70% heal without strictures).

Complete ruptures should undergo deferred primary anastomosis treatment by appropriate surgeon, managed with temporary SPC and antibiotics.

Penetrating injuries require urgent exploration:

- small defects can treated by spatulation of both ends and primary anastomosis
- longer defects may require staged repair with temporary SPC

Penile fracture related injuries can be repaired by simple closure or primary anastomosis.

POSTERIOR URETHRAL INJURIES

Posterior injuries happen most commonly in situations of trauma and are prioritised accordingly.

Single gentle attempt at urethral catheterisation is permissible and excludes significant urethral injury if easily successful.

SPC (under US guidance) urinary diversion is desirable as it allows:

- urine output monitoring
- avoids painful retention
- minimise extravasation and thus subsequent infection

The timing of surgical intervention is classified as:

- immediate: < 48 hours from injury
- delayed primary: 2 days – 2 weeks from injury
- deferred: > 3 months from injury

Partial Ruptures

Can be managed with urethral catheter or SPC in situ for > 4 weeks.

Repeat urethography is essential prior to removing catheter.

Subsequent strictures can be managed by urethrotomy if small / short, or anastomotic urethroplasty if long / dense.

Complete Rupture

Options for timing of surgical repair include *immediate, delayed primary* or *deferred*.

Deferred repair is preferred in specialist centres in the UK because it allows:
- patient to recover from major trauma (likely to allow lithotomy position)
- pelvic haematoma / urinary extravasation reduction (urethral ends come closer together, reducing length of defect and need for mobilisation during primary anastomosis)
- prostate descend to normal position following haematoma resolution
- reduction in poor outcomes

Deferred repair necessitates > 3 months of prior SPC urinary diversion.

Most PFUDDs are short and treated with one-stage perineal anastomotic repair.

Scar tissue is excised, both healthy urethral ends are spatulated with the key objective of achieving <u>tension-free anastomosis.</u>

Stricture rates are 10%.

Immediate urethroplasty is not recommended and should not be performed due to high rates of strictures (70%), incontinence (20%) and ED (40%).

This is because visualisation due to haematoma is poor, which does permit accurate assessment of the urethral defect and thus need for debridement.

Early realignment is only advisable in presence of concomitant bladder neck and / or rectal injury.

Bladder neck injury with PFUDD will lead to incontinence without surgical repair.

Early realignment performed endoscopically with cystoscopy-guided wire insertion over which a catheter is passed and left in situ > 4 weeks.

Open realignment is an alternative option.

In cases featuring a significant loss of length, the urethra requires mobilisation to allow it to stretch and achieve a tension-free anastomosis.

This can be achieved by:

1. separating crura at base of penis (where they first come together and run alongside, potential space until the 5–7cm distal to the base where they fuse)
2. spatulate dorsal ends and suture skin / buccal mucosa for anastomosis

FEMALE URETHRAL INJURY

Urethral injuries in females are very rare and pelvic fractures are main aetiological cause.

Usually longitudinal tear of anterior wall associated with vaginal laceration.

Urethral injury in females in context of pelvic fracture should be suspected with blood at vaginal introitus, visible haematuria, urinary retention and / or labial swelling.

Distal injuries can be left un-repaired as no disruption to continence mechanism.

Primary suturing of urethral ends can be performed retro-pubically (proximal injury) or trans-vaginally (mid-urethral injury).

METASTATIC SPINAL CORD COMPRESSION

Defined as spinal cord compression (SCC) by direct pressure and / or vertebral collapse by metastases or direct extension of malignancy that threatens neurological disability.

EPIDEMIOLOGY

Majority of urological related cases are due to prostate cancer.

Only 2 / 3 of patients presenting with SCC will recover any function within one month, if presenting unable to stand or walk.

95% of patients will complain of back and / or nerve root pain and have positive bone scan.

20% have multi-level spinal metastatic infiltration.

DIAGNOSTIC EVALUATION

Patient history should enquire specifically regarding:
- neurological symptom onset, duration and progression
- red flag symptoms including night-time pain, pain lying flat
- urological history for prostate cancer and latest PSA
- previous spinal pathology / surgery

Patient examination should include:
- full peripheral neurological examination of lower limbs
- anal tone and sensation (S2–4)

Imaging modality of choice is emergency full MRI of the spine with contrast.

MANAGEMENT

The patient should be resuscitated in a systematic Airway to Exposure fashion with a multi-disciplinary approach (orthopaedics, oncology, palliative care).

The local MSCC co-ordinator should be informed.

Patient should be nursed flat with neutral spine alignment.

Initial treatment involves high-dose corticosteroids (e.g. dexamethasone) +/- PPI cover.

Hormone therapy for castration can be commenced if known prostate cancer or very high PSA.

Definitive treatment includes fractionated targeted radiotherapy to the spine, or urgent neurosurgical spinal decompression.

PENILE FRACTURE

EPIDEMIOLOGY

Penile fracture is most common form of blunt penile trauma.

Sexual intercourse most common cause (50%), may occur in masturbation and rolling over in bed.

Penile fracture is more likely if sexual partner is on top.

5–10% of cases of penile fracture have an associated urethral injury. [4]

AETIOLOGY

The fracture is due to the rupture of the tunica albuginea (TA) of the erect penis.

The TA is 2mm thick in flaccid state but thins to 0.25mm during erection and is therefore more vulnerable to rupture if penis is forcibly bent.

Ventral TA is thinnest area and penile fracture are most common in this area.

DIAGNOSTIC EVALUATION

Diagnosis of penile fracture is clinical and based on history and examination findings, however further investigations can aid locate the fracture site and surgical planning.

Patient *history* should address in particular:
- nature of precipitating event (vigorous sex, position)
- sudden onset penile pain associated with popping sounds
- rapid detumescence of penis following injury
- any blood per urethra

Patient *examination* may reveal:
- penile bruising and swelling to resemble aubergine
- bruising to perineum, scrotum and lower abdominal wall (ruptured Buck's fascia)
- palpable defect of TA over site of tear
- stigmata of urethral injury, including blood per meatus, painful voiding, retention of urine

IMAGING

US of penis is readily available and can detect site of TA tear and overlying haematoma.

MRI is accurate investigation and can detect even small tears of the TA (the penis should be taped to the lower abdominal wall during the scan).

Urethrogram may be used to evaluate urethral injury; this can be done pre-operatively or on table.

Cavernosography is rarely used, as it is associated with priapism and risk of corporal fibrosis.

MANAGEMENT

Early surgical exploration (within 24 hours from injury) is recommended and TA repair is considered the treatment of choice.

Conservative treatment (ice, anti-inflammatories, abstinence from sex) is associated with higher incidence of penile fibrosis, erectile dysfunction and penile curvature.

SURGICAL REPAIR

Patient is adequately consented, anaesthetised and prepped supine on the operating table with all components of the WHO Surgical Checklist complete:

- gently pass a 12F urethral catheter, if this is easy then the patient does not require a cystoscopy to evaluate for urethral injury
- circumferential incision proximal to corona to de-glove the penis
- identify TA defect site and evacuate any overlying haematoma
- repair defect with 2'0 PDS interrupted (absorbable)
- any urethral injuries are to be repaired with 4'0 PDS over catheter (consider on-table retrograde urethrogram)
- may complete with circumcision

The patient is advised to abstain from sexual intercourse for ≥ 6 weeks after surgery.

Complications include penile curvature and erectile dysfunction.

PRIAPISM

Priapism is a prolonged and unwanted erection, in absence of sexual stimulus, <u>lasting > 4 hours.</u>

EPIDEMIOLOGY

Peak incidence age 5–10 years and 20–50 years

> 95% of all priapism episodes are "ischaemic".

Sickle cell disease is the most common cause in childhood accounting for > 60% of cases and > 20% of adults (lifetime risk in sickle cell patients is 1 / 3 approx).

PATHOPHYSIOLOGY

Ischaemic priapism > 4 hours is considered the same as compartment syndrome.

Histological changes noted in priapism include:
- interstitial oedema
- progressive destruction of sinusoidal epithelium
- exposure of basement membrane after 24 hours
- smooth muscle necrosis with fibrosis after 48 hours

Emergency medical intervention is required to prevent the irreversible changes of necrosis and fibrosis which can cause permanent ED.

The duration of priapism is the most significant predictor for development of ED.

CLASSIFICATION

The two common types of priapism are *ischaemic* (low-flow) and *non-ischaemic* (high-flow).

A less common type is *stuttering* (recurrent) priapism.

ISCHAEMIC (LOW-FLOW)

Ischaemic priapism occurs due to veno-occlusion (intra-cavernosal pressures > 80mmHg).

This is the most common form (> 95%).

Characterised by a painful and rigid erection, with low / absent cavernosal blood flow which requires emergency intervention.

Blood gas shows hypoxia, acidosis and appears dark in colour.

NON-ISCHAEMIC (HIGH-FLOW)

Non-ischaemic priapism occurs due to unregulated arterial flow.

Presents as painless and semi-rigid erection.

Usually due to previous trauma and subsequent fistula formation, blood gas is similar to arterial blood and condition usually self-limiting.

RECURRENT (STUTTERING)

Usually seen in sickle cell disease.

Commonly high-flow type of priapism (can also be low-flow), and management relies on optimising the underlying haematological condition.

AETIOLOGY

Priapism can be primary (idiopathic) in nature.

Secondary causes of priapism include:
- intra-cavernosal injections: papaverine > PGE-1
- PDE5i drugs: not a risk factor per se, however carefully counsel sickle cell patients
- haematological: leukaemia, sickle cell disease
- trauma: resulting in A-V fistula formation
- infective: malaria, rabies, genito-urinary sepsis
- oncological: infiltrating pelvic malignancy

DIAGNOSTIC EVALUATION

Main aims of history and examination are to identify aetiological cause and sub-type of priapism.

PATIENT HISTORY

The key points in taking the history of priapism include:
- time of onset of erection and presence / absence of sexual stimulus

- presence of pain
- previous similar episode and their treatment
- drug history to include ED-treatment medication
- history of pelvic trauma, known malignancy, sickle cell disease

PATIENT EXAMINATION

A systematic Airway to Exposure assessment of the patient is recommended, providing analgesia.

The following particular areas are to be examined:

- abdomen – for palpable masses / organomegaly suggesting malignancy
- penis – rigid tender corpora with soft glans (low-flow)
- DRE – palpate for advanced pelvic malignancy

BASELINE INVESTIGATIONS

Blood tests should be performed to assess FBC, differential white cell count, platelet count and coagulation profile to assess anaemia and haematological malignancies.

Aspirate blood from corpora using large butterfly needle:

- ischaemic priapism will yield acidotic result with high pCO_2
- non-ischaemic priapism will yield similar gas result to normal arterial blood

IMAGING

Routine imaging is not required to distinguish between low vs. high flow priapism.

Penile colour Doppler US of the penis can be used as an adjunct or alternative to blood gas analysis for differentiation between low vs. high flow priapism

- ischaemic priapism reveals little / no flow in cavernosal arteries and corpora
- non-ischaemic shows high-peak systolic velocities (possible fistula)

The role of MRI is controversial – it may help evaluating cases of prolonged ischaemic priapism as to the viability of the corpora and presence of penile fibrosis.

MANAGEMENT (LOW-FLOW)

Acute ischaemic priapism is a medical emergency and urgent intervention is mandatory.

The aim of any treatment is to restore penile flaccidity to prevent damage to corpora.

First line treatments for priapism > 4 hours are recommended prior to any surgical intervention, conversely symptoms > 72 hours imply that such treatments would be futile.

Sickle cell patients require oxygenation, rehydration and liaising with haematologist.

ASPIRATION OF CORPORA

Consider a penile block with 10ml of 1% lidocaine (if pain is issue).

Insert large gauge butterfly needle into corpora cavernosa via side of the penis (some insert one either side to allow for irrigation and drainage).

Aspirate stagnant blood to drain corpora – flush syringe with normal saline. Do not aspirate more than 100–150mL of blood; detumescence is expected with this amount drained.

This process should be continued until draining fresh red blood and detumescence achieved.

Success rate is 30% with aspiration alone.

INTRA-CAVERNOSAL PHENYLEPHRINE

If aspiration has been unsuccessful, keep butterfly in situ and prepare phenylephrine.

Phenylephrine is the drug of choice due to high selectivity for α-1 adrenergic receptor, however due to potential cardio-vascular side effects the patient should be in monitored setting.

Dilute to 500µg / mL (i.e. dilute 10mg in 20mL saline) and give 0.5mL every 5 minutes into corpora.

Maximum dosage is 1mg within one hour.

An alternative option is metaraminol (also α-1 adrenergic receptor agonist) however this is not first choice agent as greater potential for cardiovascular side effects.

Consider *terbutaline* (PO) as an adjunct medication in priapism caused by intra-cavernosal injections (e.g. prostaglandins).

SURGICAL INTERVENTION

Surgery in the form of penile shunt surgery should only be considered when 1st line treatments have failed (ideally > 1 hour of treatment attempts).

Shunt surgery aims to provide exit for ischaemic blood from corpora to restore normal circulation.

It is conventional for distal shunt procedures to be tried before proximal shunting.

Erectile recovery in priapism > 36 hours low even with shunt procedures (ie. consider prosthesis)

Winter Shunt (Distal)

Insert Trucut biopsy needle to create fistula between glans and each corpora.

Easy to perform (however reportedly least successful procedure)

Ebbehoj Technique (Distal)

Multiple tunica incision windows between glans and each tip of corpora using blade

T-Shunt (Distal)

Bilateral procedure, place scalpel vertically through glans lateral to meatus into corpora, then rotate this by 90° and pull out.

Al-Ghorab Procedure (Distal)

Open procedure consisting of open bilateral excision of cone segments of distal tunica albuginea, along with subsequent glans closure with absorbable sutures

Proximal Shunts

Quackle's technique and Grayhack's procedure are recognised proximal shunts.

PRIAPISM

The overall efficacy of shunt procedures is questionable – likely high rates of ED.

No particular shunting technique is known to be superior than the others.

Consider an intra-operative smooth muscle biopsy to prove necrosis, which can have medico-legal implications as well as direct management for prosthesis.

PENILE PROSTHESIS INSERTION

Prolonged ischaemic priapism will lead to necrosis, fibrosis with penile induration and shortening.

The resulting ED is likely to be permanent and refractory to medical therapy.

Recommended to insert prosthesis early, in cases of severe and prolonged ischaemic priapism, as insertion later with fibrosis is very challenging with poor outcomes.

A malleable prosthesis should be inserted first, to be changed to inflatable one later on.

There are no clear indications when to insert prosthesis, however relative indications include:
- prolonged ischaemic priapism > 36 hours
- smooth muscle biopsy proven necrosis
- failure of aspiration, phenylephrine and shunting surgery
- MRI evidence of fibrosis

MANAGEMENT (HIGH-FLOW)

The most frequent cause of high-flow priapism is blunt groin trauma.

Trauma leads to laceration of cavernosal artery leading to high-flow fistula between artery and sinusoidal tissue, which is unregulated and leads to erection.

Patient history may report local trauma, non-painful erections and sexual function possible.

Examination will reveal semi-rigid erection.

Corporal aspiration will reveal bright red blood with readings similar to arterial blood.

Management of high-flow priapism is not an emergency because the penis is not ischaemic – therefore aspiration is not mandatory as matter of urgency.

Request Penile Doppler US which may reveal fistula.

Selective arteriography can confirm site of injury.

Patient can be discharged home after investigations and confirmation of diagnosis.

- many can be managed conservatively
- selective embolisation is an option for those wanting treatment (use autologous clot or fat)
- open ligation is rare

Anti-androgens (e.g. bicalutamide) can be used, but only in adults.

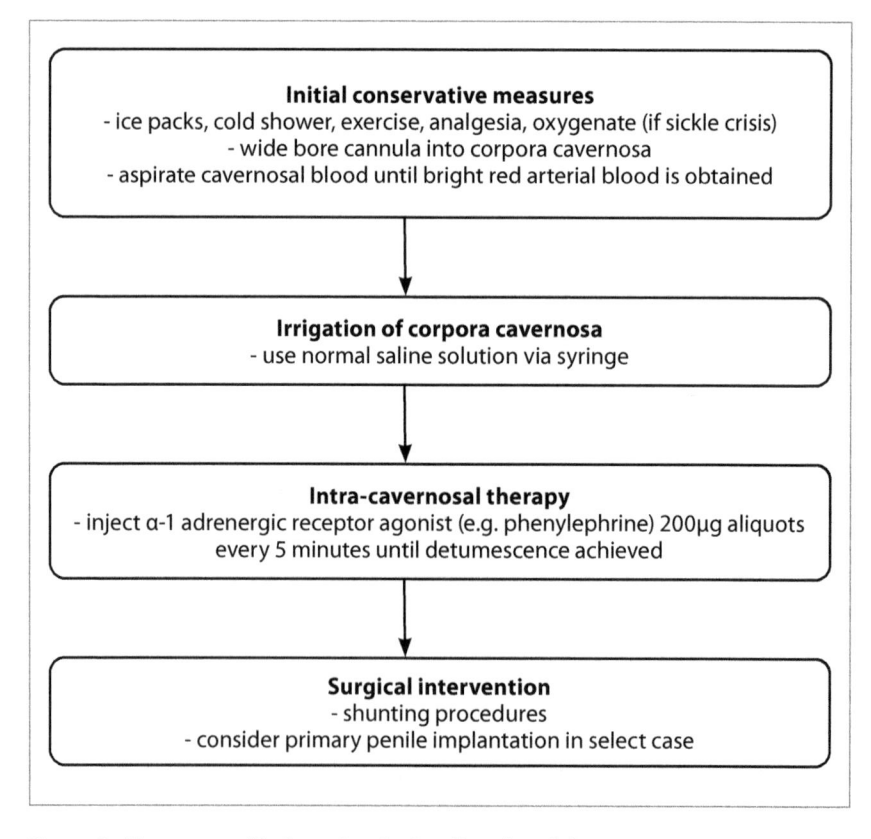

```
┌─────────────────────────────────────────────────────────────┐
│              Initial conservative measures                  │
│   - ice packs, cold shower, exercise, analgesia,            │
│     oxygenate (if sickle crisis)                            │
│   - wide bore cannula into corpora cavernosa                │
│   - aspirate cavernosal blood until bright red              │
│     arterial blood is obtained                              │
└─────────────────────────────────────────────────────────────┘
                            │
                            ▼
┌─────────────────────────────────────────────────────────────┐
│              Irrigation of corpora cavernosa                │
│             - use normal saline solution via syringe        │
└─────────────────────────────────────────────────────────────┘
                            │
                            ▼
┌─────────────────────────────────────────────────────────────┐
│                  Intra-cavernosal therapy                   │
│   - inject α-1 adrenergic receptor agonist                  │
│     (e.g. phenylephrine) 200μg aliquots                     │
│     every 5 minutes until detumescence achieved             │
└─────────────────────────────────────────────────────────────┘
                            │
                            ▼
┌─────────────────────────────────────────────────────────────┐
│                   Surgical intervention                     │
│                   - shunting procedures                     │
│   - consider primary penile implantation in select case     │
└─────────────────────────────────────────────────────────────┘
```

Figure 2 – Treatment of ischaemic priapism flowchart [5]

SEPSIS, ANAPHYLAXIS AND BIOCHEMICAL EMERGENCIES

SYSTEMIC INFLAMMATORY RESPONSE SYNDROME

Systemic Inflammatory Response Syndrome (SIRS) is the response of the body to both infectious and non-infectious stimuli.

SIRS is an inflammatory state which may feature both pro- and anti-inflammatory components.

Sepsis may lead to SIRS, as well as non-infectious stimuli such as burns, pancreatitis and trauma.

Criteria for diagnosis of SIRS are listed [Table 6] – at least 2 of the criteria must be present.

Table 6 – the SIRS criteria [6]

Temperature	> 38°C or < 36°C
Heart Rate	> 90 / minute
Respiratory Rate	> 20 / minute or PaCO2 < 32 mmHg (< 4.3 kPa)
	or need for mechanical ventilation
WCC	< 4 x 10^9/L or > 12 x 10^9/L
	or > 10% presence of immature neutrophils

SEPSIS DEFINITIONS

Sepsis, proven infection causing a SIRS

Severe sepsis, sepsis associated with hypotension, organ hypo-perfusion and dysfunction, leading to lactic acidosis, oliguria or alteration in mental state.

Septic shock, sepsis with hypotension despite fluid resuscitation along with end-organ hypo-perfusion leading to lactic acidosis, oliguria or alteration in mental state

Refractory septic shock, resistant to fluid resuscitation and pharmacological intervention

SEPSIS-6 CARE BUNDLE PROTOCOL

Patients can be systematically resuscitated in an Airway to exposure fashion, and in particular to sepsis according to the sepsis 6 care bundle protocol.

Sepsis-6 has 3 components IN (oxygen, fluids, antibiotics) and 3 OUT (catheter, lactate, cultures).

Table 7 – the sepsis-6 bundle [7]

Sepsis-6 Component	Notes
Oxygen (IN)	15 L / minute via non-rebreathe mask
IV Fluids (IN)	Large bore IV access, 1000ml Hartmann's bolus
Antibiotics (IN)	Broad-spectrum according to local guidelines
Monitor urine output (OUT)	Insert urinary catheter and monitor urine output hourly
Lactate (OUT)	Obtained from blood sample
Blood cultures (OUT)	Obtained from blood sample

qSOFA SCORE [8]

The quick sepsis related organ failure assessment (qSOFA) is a bedside prompt to aid identification of patients with suspected infection who are at greater risk of poorer outcome outside ITU.

The components of the qSOFA score:

- low blood pressure (systolic 100mmHg)
- raised respiratory rate (22 / minute)
- altered mental state (GCS < 15)

SOFA SCORE [9]

An alternative scoring system for sepsis is the sequential organ failure assessment score (SOFA):

- respiratory (PaO_2)
- cardiovascular (MAP)
- renal (urine output or creatinine)
- coagulation (platelet count)

- neurology (GCS)
- liver (bilirubin)

Used to monitor a patient's stay on ITU, assessing organ system function, to predict clinical outcomes.

ANAPHYLAXIS

Management of anaphylaxis for the urologist:
- secure patient airway, give high flow oxygen, obtain IV access and place cardiac monitoring
- give 0.5mL of 1:1000 adrenaline (IM) (i.e. 500mcg)
- give 10mg of chlorphenamine (IV) + 200mg of hydrocortisone (IV)
- request immediate help via EMRT call

BIOCHEMICAL EMERGENCIES

HYPERKALAEMIA

Obtain ECG – possible changes include tall tented T-waves, wide QRS complex.

Management of hyperkalaemia for the urologist:
1. Protect myocardium – 10mL of 10% calcium gluconate
2. Drive K^+ into cells – 10units of actrapid in 50mL of 50% glucose + 5mg salbutamol (neb)
3. Deplete total body K^+ – calcium resonium 15mg (PO) TDS

Ensure ECG is repeated if changes were noted on initial trace, consider cardiac monitoring.

Regularly re-check K^+ (and blood sugar) until this has come down into safe range.

Persisting hyperkalaemia despite medical therapy should prompt contact with on call renal medicine to consider requirement for emergency dialysis.

HYPERCALCAEMIA

Features – confusion / altered GCS / coma, thirst / dehydration, muscle weakness, arrhythmias.

Obtain ECG – possible change includes shortened QT interval.

Urgent treatment is required if Ca^{2+} > 3.0mmol/L (check PTH, albumin and renal function).

Management of hypercalcaemia for the urologist:

1. Aggressive rehydration – 4–6L of 0.9% saline (IV) over 24 hours (consider loop diuretic if patient is overloaded)
2. Bisphosphonates (IV) e.g. zoledronic acid 4mg
3. Treat underlying cause e.g. thiazide diuretics, rhabdomyolysis

Persisting hypercalcaemia despite medical therapy should prompt contact with on call renal medicine to consider requirement for emergency dialysis.

Equation for corrected calcium = (measured total Ca^{2+}) + 0.02(40 – serum albumin)

TESTICULAR TORSION

Testicular torsion is a twist of the spermatic cord, resulting in strangulation of the blood supply to the testis and epididymis.

EPIDEMIOLOGY

Testicular torsion can occur at any age, however the incidence has a bi-modal distribution with the main peak around puberty (12–18 years) and smaller peak in first year of life.

CLASSIFICATION

EXTRA-VAGINAL TORSION

Most commonly seen in the first year of life (can occur pre- or post-natally)

Incomplete fixation of gubernaculum to scrotal wall, resulting in entire testis and tunica vaginalis twisting in vertical axis on the spermatic cord, outside the tunica vaginalis

INTRA-VAGINAL TORSION

Most common form of testicular torsion seen in adolescents

Usually due to congenital *bell-clapper deformity*, whereby the testis not attached posteriorly to inner scrotum by the mesorchium such that it is free-floating and can rotate more readily

DIAGNOSTIC EVALUATION

Patient *history* should enquire in particular regarding:
- time / nature / activity at the onset of pain (often waking from sleep)
- any previous similar self-limiting episodes (to suggest intermittent torsion)
- any previous scrotal surgery or exploration

Patient *examination* should evaluate:
- tender affected testicle (rather than just superior pole, suggesting torted hydatid)
- absent cremasteric reflex (sensitivity close to 100%, specificity 66%)
- high-riding and horizontal lie testis

- mild fever
- elevation of testicle does not ameliorate symptoms (negative Prehn's sign)

Urine dipstick test is usually normal in testicular torsion.

Cremasteric Reflex

Elicited by stroking the inner surface of the thigh in males – immediate contraction of the cremaster muscle that draws ipsilateral testis superiorly

Sensory – stimulation of ilio-inguinal nerve

Motor – activation of genital branch of the genito-femoral nerve

IMAGING

Testicular torsion is a clinical diagnosis and the gold-standard management for suspected testicular torsion is urgent scrotal exploration.

The use of radiological investigations should not delay patient transfer to theatre.

Doppler colour US, has a role in patients where clinical features are equivocal and there is no clinical indication for urgent exploration.

$$\text{sensitivity} < 90\% \text{ and specificity} < 95\%$$

US is operator dependent, arterial flow can be misleading in early cases of torsion and persisting arterial flow does not exclude the diagnosis of torsion.

Radio-nuclide scanning of scrotum (using technetium-99m) is most accurate imaging technique to detect reduced radio-isotope uptake, however time-consuming and not readily available.

MANAGEMENT

Urgent surgical exploration is gold-standard and should be undertaken whenever there is clinical suspicion of testicular torsion.

The two most important determinants for testicular salvage are:
- time between symptom onset and surgical de-torsion
- degree of cord twisting (worse if > 360° rotation)

Salvage rates correlate with number of hours after onset of pain.

Testicular fixation should be performed on affected testicle (if viable) with 3'0 prolene using 3-point technique (medial, lateral, antero-inferior).

Contra-lateral fixation should be performed if testicular torsion if found or thought to have been highly likely on initial patient history and examination.

Insertion of prosthesis is not advised at time of orchidectomy due to risk of erosion.

IMPACT ON FERTILITY

The impact on fertility of testicular torsion remains unclear and evidence is conflicting.

Early surgical intervention with detorsion is likely to preserve fertility.

If testicular torsion is not treated urgently and testicle undergoes infarction, there is a risk of abscess / sinus formation, and breakdown of blood-testis barrier with subsequent risk of infertility.

Blood-testis Barrier (BTB)

BTB is a barrier between blood vessels and Sertoli cells of seminiferous tubules, formed by tight / adherens / gap junctions by intra-cellular adhesion molecules.

BTB serves to control environment in which germ cells develop (e.g. blocks entry cytotoxic agents).

If BTB is breached, sperm may enter bloodstream and immune system mounts auto-immune response against the unique sperm antigens only expressed by these cells.

The anti-sperm antibodies may bind to sperm and reduce fertility.

TUR SYNDROME

TUR syndrome is a multi-factorial syndrome arising from the absorption of large volumes of irrigation fluid (1.5% glycine) during endoscopic procedures (typically TURP).

EPIDEMIOLOGY

Incidence of 1–2% following TURP (although likely lower incidence with modern technology)

Typically TURP, however it may occur during TURBT and PCNL.

AETIOLOGY

During TURP there is 20 mL / minute fluid absorption (i.e. 1.2 L per hour) directly into peri-prostatic venous plexus (delayed absorption in retro-peritoneal and peri-vesical spaces).

1.5% glycine is hypo-tonic with respect to plasma (plasma ~ 280mmol/L, glycine ~ 220mmol/L).

Glycine is dealt with in the body as follows: [10]

[Liver]: (90%)   glycine ➡ ammonia + glycolic acid + H2O (lowers Na^+ concentration)

[Kidney]: (10%) glycine ➡ atrial natriuretic peptide (ANP)

The 3 main factors underlying the clinical symptoms of TUR syndrome include:

1. Dilutional hyponatraemia
2. Fluid overload
3. Effects of glycine toxicity

1. DILUTIONAL HYPO-NATRAEMIA

Hypo-tonic glycine in bloodstream leads to osmotic shift of water from plasma into the brain causing confusion, nausea, reduced GCS, coma, cerebral herniation and death.

Glycine also induces osmotic diuresis and loss of sodium, further exacerbated by ANP natriuresis.

Table 8 – symptoms noted with lowering concentrations of serum sodium

Sodium concentration (mmol / L)	Symptoms
130–135	Asymptomatic
120–130	Restlessness, confusion
115–120	Nausea
< 115	Seizures, coma

2. FLUID OVERLOAD

Pulmonary oedema by fluid oedema results in SOB, cyanosis and hypertension.

Later features include bradycardia and marked systolic hypotension.

3. GLYCINE TOXICITY

Glycine is inhibitory neurotransmitter in the retina – excess glycine slows down impulses from retina to cerebral cortex, which may manifest as flashing lights.

Glycine results in bradycardia due to cardio-toxic effects.

MANAGEMENT

TUR syndrome management can be divided into prevention, recognition and treatment.

Before any patient is considered for TURP, they have to be deemed fit from anaesthetic point of view and any low sodium is diagnosed and treated before surgery.

PREVENTION

The following strategies can be employed to reduce the risk of TUR syndrome:
- *operative time*, limited to < 60 minutes (consider staged procedures)
- *gland size selection*, where < 45g prostate is considered favourable
- *bipolar resection*, which uses normal saline as the irrigation fluid
- *reduce height* of irrigation bag

- *spinal anaesthesia (SA)*, allows earlier recognition based on patient symptoms

If procedure is inevitably prolonged, the anaesthetist should be asked to administer furosemide.

RECOGNITION

All TURPs should be performed under spinal anaesthesia whenever medically safe and patient wishes respected.

Spinal anaesthesia allows assessment of mental state, nausea, flashing lights and malaise.

General anaesthesia signs include hypertension due to fluid overload (early) or arrhythmias and bradycardia (late).

(Addition of 1% ethanol in irrigant allows alcohol breath level monitoring to estimate volume of excess absorbed fluid.)

TREATMENT

Intra-operative recognition mandates termination of procedure as soon as safely possible.

Mild cases: give 40mg IV furosemide (causes loss of more water than sodium)

close observation

repeat UEs

inform critical care out-reach

Severe cases: give 40mg IV furosemide

immediate critical care out-reach review and transfer to high-dependency

invasive BP monitoring, central line insertion, intubation, consider mannitol

Hyponatraemia correction aimed at < 1 mmol / L / hour to avoid central pontine myelinolysis.

COMPONENTS OF COMMON IV FLUIDS:

Normal saline – 154mmol/L Na^+ + 154mmol/L Cl^-

1.5% glycine – 15g of glycine per litre

Hartmann's – 131mmol/L Na^+ + 111mmol/L Cl^- + 29mmol/L HCO_3^- + 5mmol/L K^+ + 2mmol/L CA^{2+}

5% glucose – 278mmol/L glucose (50g)

URETHRAL STRICTURES

A urethral stricture is scar in sub-epithelial tissues of corpus spongiosum which results in narrowing of the lumen of the urethra.

Only anterior urethra is surrounded by corpus spongiosum, therefore true strictures can only affect the anterior urethra (posterior narrowing is termed stenosis).

AETIOLOGY

The scar tissue in the spongy erectile tissue of the corpus spongiosum arise from:

- inflammatory processes, e.g. gonococcal urethritis, BXO
- trauma, particularly straddle injuries
- iatrogenic, such as traumatic catheterisation, TUR surgery, prostate cancer surgery
- idiopathic, (often contain high levels of smooth muscle on biopsy)

DIAGNOSTIC EVALUATION

Patient history should specifically address the following:

- duration and onset of urinary symptoms
- previous urological history / interventions / operations
- previous trauma or straddle injuries
- previous STIs

Patient examination is often unremarkable, however one must assess for visible signs of BXO.

Further investigation involves uroflowmetry, flexible urethroscopy or retrograde urethrogram (RU)

In uroflowmetry the patient is asked to void > 150mL of urine onto flow-rate meter.

Classical pattern with stricture is plateau-shaped, with little change in flow rate [see following trace].

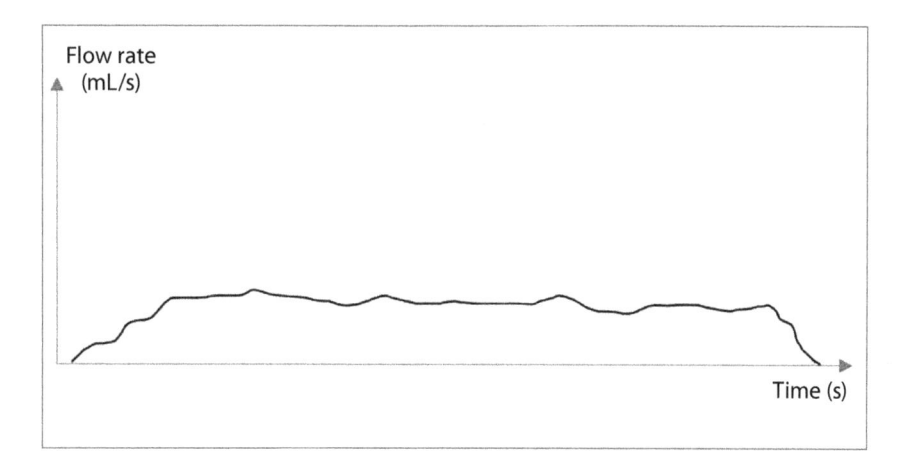

Figure 3 – Typical uroflowmetry trace of urethral stricture

Flexible cystoscopy allows direct visualisation of the stricture.

RU in specialist centres is performed instead of flexible urethroscopy as it provides more detailed information about the urethra (length and number of strictures).

US useful to detect bladder thickening suggesting chronic outflow obstruction and residual urine

MANAGEMENT

SHORT STRICTURES

A newly diagnosed short (< 2 cm) urethral stricture in a patient who is a fit candidate for anaesthesia should be referred for surgical intervention.

Options include optical urethrotomy vs. urethral dilatation (no advantage in outcomes).

Urethral dilatation is preferable for strictures close to sphincter mechanism.

A catheter should be kept in-situ for 3 days and patient referred for intermittent self-dilatation (ISD) teaching for 6 months.

The complications of urethrotomy [shown below] include 50% recurrence rate (and 90% after treatment of recurrent stricture).

DE-NOVO SHORT STRICTURES

For recurrent strictures a patient should be considered for anastomotic bulbar urethroplasty.

The pre-requisites for anastomotic bulbar urethroplasty include:
- recurrent short bulbar stricture < 2cm in length
- pelvic-fracture related injury (distraction rather than stricture)
- not appropriate for more distal penile strictures as will result in penile deformity on erection

Any anastomotic repair must be spatulated, <u>tension-free</u> and catheterised.

Curative in 90% at 10 years follow up

Complications include post-micturition dribble (division of bulbo-spongiosus) and recurrence.

LONG STRICTURES

For long bulbar strictures not amenable to anastomotic bulbar urethroplasty, alternative option is *substitution* urethroplasty.

Dorsal stricturotomy is performed with placement of a dorsal patch (Barbagli procedure) using a buccal mucosal graft.

Success rates are inferior – 85% patency rates at 3 years deteriorating at 5% yearly such that by 10 years approximately half the patients develop recurrence.

This is not appropriate for radiotherapy strictures as grafts will not take (i.e. genital skin flap).

BUCCAL MUCOSA

This is the graft of choice in substitution urethroplasty because:
- readily available in sufficient quantity
- minimal morbidity to donor site
- accustomed to wet environment
- resistant to skin diseases
- anti-microbial properties
- behaves like full-thickness graft and thus takes well

Graft-take will take approximately 96 hours.

Initial process undergoes two phases:

- *imbibition*, graft obtains nutrients from host bed (graft temperature below core body)
- *inosculation*, phase in which true micro-circulation is re-established in graft

A successful graft will re-establish its blood supply by revascularisation.

Buccal mucosa has pan-laminar plexus, allowing it to be thinned during harvesting.

Dorsal placement of patch preferred as well-supported by cavernous bodies, preventing outpouching.

Full thickness grafts include both dermis and epidermis, are however less likely to take as they are thicker than partial thickness grafts and rely on less robust sub-dermal plexus.

Partial thickness skin grafts are deficient in collagen, therefore will contract and inferior cosmetically.

REFERENCES

1. https://www.aast.org/library/traumatools/injuryscoringscales.aspx#blatter [last accessed 23 May 2020].
2. Kitrey ND, Djakovic N, Kuehhas FE, et al. (2018) EAU Guidelines on Urological Trauma. Available at: https://uroweb.org/wp-content/uploads/EAU-Guidelines-on-Urological-Trauma-2018-large-text.pdf [last accessed 23 May 2020].
3. Sharma DM, Shergill IS, Arya M. Urological emergencies, Part 2. In: Arya M, Shergill IS, Fernando HS, et al. (2018) Viva Practice for the FRCS (Urol) and Postgraduate Urology Examinations, 2nd Edition, CRC Press, London.
4. Amer T, Wilson R, Chlosta P, et al. (2016). Penile fracture: a meta-analysis. *Urologia internationalis*, 96(3), 315–329.
5. Hatzimouratidis K, Giuliano F, Moncada I. et al. (2018) EAU Guidelines on Erectile Dysfunction, Premature Ejaculation, Penile Curvature and Priapism. Available at: https://uroweb.org/wp-content/uploads/EAU-Guidelines-on-Male-Sexual-Dysfunction-2018-large-text.pdf [last accessed 24 May 2020].
6. Comstedt P, Storgaard M, Lassen AT. (2009) The Systemic Inflammatory Response Syndrome (SIRS) in acutely hospitalised medical patients: a cohort study. *Scandinavian journal of trauma, resuscitation and emergency medicine*, 17(1), 67.
7. The College of Emergency Medicine, "Sepsis". Available at: https://www.rcem.ac.uk/docs/Sepsis/Sepsis%20Toolkit.pdf [last accessed 24 May 2020].
8. Marik PE, Taeb AM. (2017) SIRS, qSOFA and new sepsis definition. *Journal of thoracic disease*, 9(4), 943.
9. Jones AE, Trzeciak S, Kline JA. (2009) The Sequential Organ Failure Assessment score for predicting outcome in patients with severe sepsis and evidence of hypoperfusion at the time of emergency department presentation. *Critical care medicine*, 37(5), 1649.
10. Shergill IS, Jameel B. Urological Emergencies, Part 1. In: In: Arya M, Shergill IS, Fernando HS, et al. (2018) Viva Practice for the FRCS (Urol) and Postgraduate Urology Examinations, 2nd Edition, CRC Press, London.

EMERGENCY UROLOGY MCQS

1. Which is the most appropriate choice of suture to repair the tunica albuginea of a ruptured testis due to traumatic injury?
   A) 2'0 vicryl
   B) 4'0 vicryl
   C) 2'0 prolene
   D) 4'0 prolene
   E) 3'0 ethilon

2. Which of the following is not a parameter that is part of the calculation of the SOFA score?
   A) GCS
   B) systolic blood pressure
   C) platelet count
   D) serum bilirubin concentration
   E) serum creatinine concentration

3. Which of the following histological changes occurs in untreated priapism?
   A) basement membrane exposure
   B) green-stained collagen with picrosirius red
   C) decrease in smooth muscle cells
   D) increase in elastic system fibres
   E) all of the above

4. By what process does a graft obtain nutrients from its host bed?
   A) diapedesis
   B) active transport
   C) inosculation
   D) infiltration
   E) imbibition

5. What is the correct dose of adrenaline to be given as emergency treatment for anaphylaxis?
   A) 0.5mL of 1:1000 adrenaline (IM)
   B) 0.5mL of 1:10000 adrenaline (IM)
   C) 1mL of 1:100 adrenaline (IM)
   D) 1mL of 1:1000 adrenaline (IM)
   E) 1mL of 1:10000 adrenaline (IM)

6. Which of the following is not an accepted indication to perform an emergency CT scan in the context of renal trauma?
    A) concomitant fracture of the lower ribs
    B) history of rapid deceleration
    C) non-visible haematuria with haemodynamic instability
    D) visible haematuria with haemodynamic stability
    E) systolic BP < 100mmHg

7. What is the most likely profile of biochemical abnormalities seen in TUR syndrome?
    A) hyperkalaemia, hyponatraemia, hyperammonaemia
    B) hypokalaemia, hyponatraemia, hyperammonaemia
    C) hyper kalaemia, hyponatraemia, hypoammonaemia
    D) hypokalaemia, hyponatraemia, hypoammonaemia
    E) none of the above

8. Which of the following is not a set parameter in the SIRS criteria scoring?
    A) temperature < 36°C
    B) $PaCO_2$ < 4.3KPa
    C) WCC > 14 x 10^9/L
    D) heart rate > 90 beats / minute
    E) presence > 10% immature neutrophils

9. Which of the following is false regarding the blood-testis barrier?
    A) formed by punctate tight junctions between Sertoli cells
    B) located on the luminal side of the basally positioned spermatogonia
    C) the formation of the barrier does not coincide with increasing numbers of spermatocytes
    D) the barrier is stabilised by espin proteins
    E) DHT induces the formation of the barrier, however FSH alone does not

10. The correct equation for calculating the corrected calcium value is:
    A) (measured total Ca^{2+})− 0.02(40 − serum albumin)
    B) (measured total Ca^{2+})− 0.02(serum albumin − 40)
    C) (measured total Ca^{2+})+ 0.02(40 − serum albumin)
    D) (measured total Ca^{2+})+ 0.02(serum albumin − 40)
    E) (measured total Ca^{2+})x 0.02(serum albumin − 40)

11. Which of the following statements regarding penile fracture in male patient is true:
    A) right sided corporal injuries are more common than left
    B) the most common site of injury to tunica albuginea is on the dorsal aspect of penis
    C) the sexual position with highest risk of penile fracture is male patient missionary on top
    D) USS may show hyper-echoic discontinuity in the normally echogenic tunica albuginea
    E) bilateral corporal injuries do not increase the risk of urethral injury

12. The correct dosage of intra-cavernosal phenylephrine to treat priapism is:
    A) 100µg every 5–10 minutes, to a maximum of 0.5mg in 1 hour
    B) 250µg every 5–10 minutes, to a maximum of 2mg in 1 hour
    C) 100mg every 5–10 minutes, to a maximum of 0.5g in 1 hour
    D) 250mg every 5–10 minutes, to a maximum of 2g in 1 hour
    E) none of the above

13. All of the following are recognised causes of priapism, except:
    A) buproprion
    B) olanzapine
    C) total parenteral nutrition
    D) peritoneal dialysis
    E) use of unfractionated heparin

14. An 8 year-old boy has a clear history of acute testicular torsion for 5 hours, and you wish to proceed to scrotal exploration. Only his father is present. He has never been married to the boy's mother and is not on the birth certificate of his son. The mother is abroad for work and cannot be contacted anytime soon.

    His father refuses consent. What is the most appropriate course of action?

    A) proceed to operate – the father has no parental rights for consent
    B) proceed to operate – evaluate whether boy is Gillick competent to consent
    C) proceed to operate – via double signature consent from consultant colleague
    D) you cannot operate – respect the father's wishes
    E) you cannot operate – apply for emergency decision by the courts

15. Regarding surgical intervention for ureteric injuries, which of the following are true:
    A) in the unstable trauma patient with on-table incidental finding of ureteric transection, the affected ureter should not be ligated
    B) Psoas hitch procedure may injure the genito-femoral nerve, as this lies on the psoas muscle
    C) Psoas hitch procedure can be aided by division of the inferior vesical pedicle
    D) Prophylactic ureteric stenting prior to complex pelvic surgery reduces rates of ureteric injury
    E) AAST Grade 3 ureteric injuries cannot be managed by stenting alone

16. Which of the following statements regarding testicular torsion is true:
    A) intra-vaginal torsion is most commonly seen in the 1st year of life
    B) relief of pain by elevating the testis suggests the cause is epididymitis (negative Prehn's sign)
    C) the bell-clapper abnormality is a malformation of the processus vaginalis
    D) the absent cremasteric reflex is determined by the ilioinguinal nerve as afferent supply, and pudendal nerve as efferent
    E) Doppler-US is the most accurate imaging technique, when clinically indicated

17. Which of the following statements regarding shunt treatments for priapism is false:
    A) Quackels procedure involves creating a shunt between corpora cavernosa and spongiosum at the level of the bulbar urethra
    B) Sacher approach involves a penoscrotal incision
    C) Greyhack procedure uses the saphenous vein anastomosed to the tunica albuginea
    D) Barry procedure uses the superficial vein of the penis anastomosed to the tunica albuginea
    E) Al-Ghorab procedure uses a dorsal sub-coronal incision

18. The most appropriate initial hormone therapy for a patient newly presenting with lower limb weakness, lower back pain and a PSA of 3500, is:
    A) Goserelin 3.6mg stat then 3.6mg every 28 days
    B) Goserelin 10.8mg stat then 10.8mg every 12 weeks
    C) Degarelix 60mg stat then 20mg every 28 days
    D) Degarelix 120mg stat then 40mg every 28 days
    E) Degarelix 240mg stat then 80mg every 28 days

19. Which of the following statements regarding Page phenomenon is false:
    A) results from external compression of the kidney
    B) hypertension is caused by activation of the renin-angiotensin-aldosterone system
    C) decapsulation of fibro-collagenous shell can treat refractory hypertension
    D) there is a clear association between renal biopsies and Page kidney
    E) they do not occur in transplanted kidneys

20. Which of the following statements regarding pharmacological treatment of priapism is false:
    A) phenylephrine is an option as an α-1 adrenergic receptor agonist
    B) bicalutamide is an option as a competitive androgen inhibitor
    C) terbutaline is an option as a β2-antagonist
    D) metaraminol is an option as an α-1 adrenergic receptor agonist
    E) none of the above

ANSWERS TO MCQS

STATION 1: UROLOGICAL ONCOLOGY 1
1. **B** – BSP (bone sialoprotein) has not been used for urothelial cancer detection
2. **A** – healthy bladder is blue / purple, note also the trigone may appear abnormal as it is a common site of low-grade inflammation
3. **B**
4. **A**
5. **D** – ipsilateral adrenal gland is T4, contralateral adrenal gland is M1
6. **C** – the CARMENA trial evaluated sunitinib, (A, D and E would all be correct if sunitinib were in the option), and note the primary end point was OS
7. **C**
8. **D**
9. **E** – time from diagnosis to treatment < 12 months
10. **A** – tumour thrombus below hepatic veins but > 2cm above renal vein orifice is level 2, most likely histology is RCC
11. **E**
12. **B**
13. **C**
14. **D** – Wallace 1 involves suturing the medial walls of spatulated ureters together, and anastomosing this conjoined segment to the proximal end of the open bowel segment
15. **A**
16. **D** – typical dose is 60 – 66Gy in 30 – 32 fractions over 6 weeks
17. **D** – patient with any metastasis were excluded, performance status included 0 – 1 only
18. **B** – only 20% are due to tuberous sclerosis
19. **E**
20. **C** – essential fact for the viva station (not many study percentages of trial studies need memorising but fair to say this is one of them)
21. **A**
22. **C** – prognosis is poor and 5-year survival is < 50%
23. **C**
24. **B** – attaches to the fibronectin receptor
25. **B** – severe hypokalaemia may occur (also remember that cobalamin = vitamin B12)

STATION 2: UROLOGICAL ONCOLOGY 2

1. **C** – cardiovascular disease is a caution, not contra-indication.
2. **A** – you must know TNM staging inside out for all the cancers, it is a guarantee that you will be asked a question on this in the MCQ and / or VIVA
3. **D**
4. **D**
5. **E** – >95% of prostate cancers are adenocarcinomas and the absent staining is for p63 (p53 is a tumour suppressing gene)
6. **C**
7. **B**
8. **B** – recall the 4 "R's" of radiobiology
9. **A**
10. **B**
11. **A**
12. **C** – note that it is percentage of cores with "clinically significant" prostate cancer
13. **E**
14. **D**
15. **D**
16. **B** – 3% are bilateral at presentation
17. **A**
18. **C**
19. **E**
20. **E** – note that TNM for testicular cancer has a N-stage for both clinical lymph nodes and lymph nodes on pathology (i.e. after RPLND), in this case the nodes were evaluated on CT alone
21. **B**
22. **B**
23. **D** – induction chemotherapy is x3 BEP (upfront is x1), majority of micro-metastasis outside the retroperitoneum are in the lung, relapse risk with vascular invasion is much higher at 48%
24. **A** – PET is advised if residual volume > 2cm
25. **A** – note it is tumour size > 4cm
26. **C**
27. **B** – if risk factors are all present, ITGCN is present in 1/3 contra-lateral testis
28. **E** – lymphoma can present on the penis as primary penile lymphoma, however it is not otherwise a known risk factor for SCC of the penis
29. **A**

30. **E** – careful as TNM classification for penile cancer only has M0/1 as M-stage
31. **C**
32. **C** – sexual intercourse is permitted provided patient uses condom
33. **D**
34. **A** – the patient falls within the low risk category
35. **B**

STATION 3: PAEDIATRIC UROLOGY

1. **C** – most common cause in females is ureterocoele
2. **B**
3. **A**
4. **A**
5. **B**
6. **E** – note that follow up DMSA is after 4 – 6 months
7. **D** – the contraceptive pill taken <u>after</u> conception has been shown to increase risk of hypospadias
8. **C**
9. **A** – in boys the ectopic orifice is never below the external sphincter
10. **E** – note that dysfunctional voiding is also known as Hinman's syndrome
11. **C**
12. **B** – horseshoe kidney has higher risk of Wilms' tumour and upper tract TCC, however not of RCC or other renal tumours
13. **B**
14. **E** – you should allow at least 3 months for the testis to drop into the scrotal sac spontaneously
15. **D**
16. **A** – if in a duplex system, a ureterocoele is always associated with the upper moiety
17. **D** – note that hyponatraemia is a common side effect if the child is not fluid restricted along with the medication, counselling should also include weight gain
18. **C** – PUV is relatively rare, and so although 20 – 50% of PUV patients may progress to ESRF, actually the overall proportion of paediatric ESRF caused by PUV alone is much lower at 17%.
19. **D**
20. **B** – the Swedish reflux study showed that antibiotic prophylaxis made no difference to boys in UTI rates and renal scarring, note that cefalexin can be used for prophylaxis however as per the BNF it is not licensed for this use.

21. **B** – 80% of UDT are palpable, only 1 in 3 retractile testes will become undescended, only 1 in 5 impalpable testes are absent
22. **A**
23. **A**
24. **E** – the processus vaginalis persists in ≤ 90% of newborns
25. **E**

STATION 4: EMERGENCY UROLOGY

1. **D** – requires a fine absorbable suture
2. **B** – cardiovascular element is mean arterial pressure (MAP) = (2(diastolic BP) + (systolic BP)) / 3
3. **E**
4. **E**
5. **A**
6. **E** – a systolic blood pressure of < 90mmHg at any time after injury warrants emergency CT scan
7. **A**
8. **C**
9. **C**
10. **C**
11. **A**
12. **E** – the maximum dose in 1 hour is 1mg
13. **D**
14. **A** – if a father has never been married to the mother, and is not on the birth certificate, he has no automatic legal rights to the child. Therefore, proceed on best interests due to time-sensitive nature of underlying pathology.
15. **B** – note that it is the division of the superior vesical pedicle which is performed in psoas hitch
16. **C**
17. **D**
18. **E**
19. **E** – lymphocoele around a transplanted kidney can cause Page phenomenon
20. **C** – terbutaline is a ß2-agonist